Jeanne Rose's
Modern Herbal

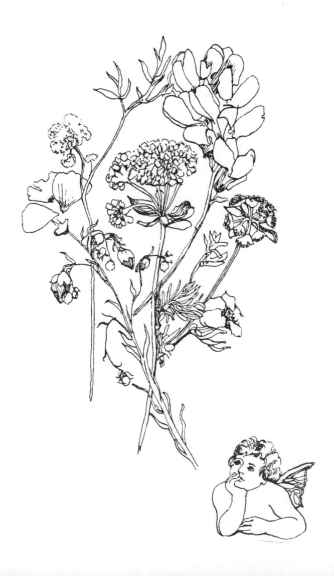

OTHER BOOKS BY JEANNE ROSE

Herbs and Things

The Herbal Body Book

Kitchen Cosmetics

Jeanne Rose's Herbal Guide to Inner Health

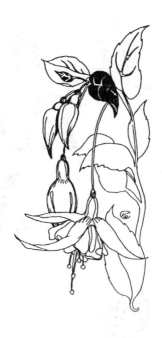

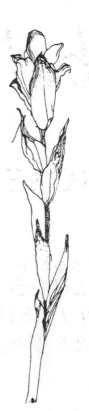

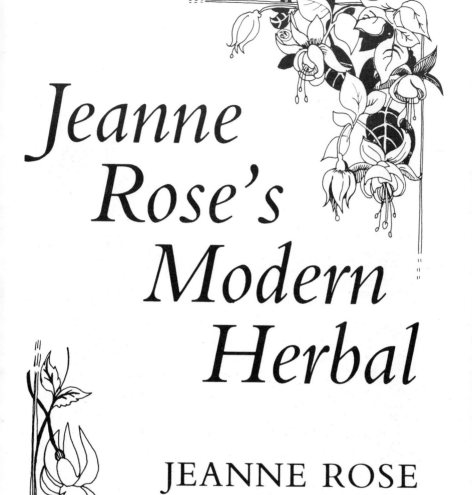

Jeanne Rose's Modern Herbal

JEANNE ROSE

Illustrated by
DIANE HALL &
CATHY DUDLEY
A Perigee Book

Perigee Books
are published by
The Putnam Publishing Group
200 Madison Avenue
New York, NY 10016

"Herbal Home Remedies," "Herbs for Modern Beauty," and "The Herbal
Pet" reprinted from The Natural Formula Book for Home and Yard,
© 1982 by Rodale Press, Inc., by permission of Rodale Press, Inc.,
Emmaus, PA 18049.
"Mothering" by Nan Ullrike Koehler, printed with permission of author.
"Homeopathic First Aid" by Dana Ullman, printed with permission of author.

Designed by Beth Tondreau Design
Typeset by Fisher Composition, Inc.

LIBRARY OF CONGRESS CATALOGING-IN-PUBLICATION DATA

Rose, Jeanne, date.
Jeanne Rose's modern herbal.

Bibliography: p.
Includes index.
1. Herbs—Therapeutic use. 2. Personal.
3. Herbs—Utilization. 4. Herbals. I. Title.
II. Title: Modern herbal.
RM666.H33R67   1987   615'.321   87-22982
ISBN 0-399-51394-9
Printed in the United States of America
1   2   3   4   5   6   7   8   9   10

PUBLISHER'S NOTE

All plants, like all medicines, may be dangerous if used improperly—if they are taken internally when prescribed for external use, if they are taken in excess, or if they are taken for too long a time. Allergic reactions and unpredictable sensitivities, particularly to douches, may develop. There are other factors to consider as well: Since the strength of wild herbs varies, knowledge of their growing conditions is helpful. Be sure your herbs are fresh and keep conditions of use as sterile as possible.

We do not advocate, endorse, or guarantee the curative effects of any of the substances listed in this book. We have made every effort to see that any botanical that is dangerous or potentially dangerous has been noted as such. When you use herbs, recognize their potency and use them with care. Medical consultation is recommended for those recipes marked as dangerous.

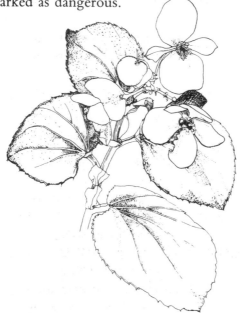

ACKNOWLEDGMENTS

Anton Mueller, my editor at Putnam; Robert Gordon, my friend and attorney; and all those herbalists who came before and are my inspiration.

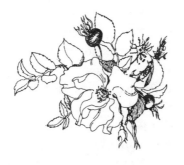

Dedicated to the Ones I Love

———— o ————

LOIS LIPPINCOTT

&

To those individuals who helped me through one of the most difficult times of my life: Lewis Lehman, M.D., who is a caring and compassionate physician; Nan Koehler, whose pure spirit and sweet nurturing nature are an inspiration; Laeh Garfield, an extraordinary psychic; and those friends who took care of me, especially Penelope deVries (she made me laugh when I couldn't), Albert Seligman and Wayne Scott (men friends, dear friends), *and* Marshall and Lauren Krause, who gave me Joel Alter, who is a healer and sleep giver *and* to Cal Bewicke and Thom Hart, who gave me work to do.

Especially to one of the sweetest, nicest kids in the world, my son, Bryan L. Moore.

Contents

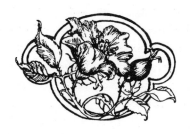

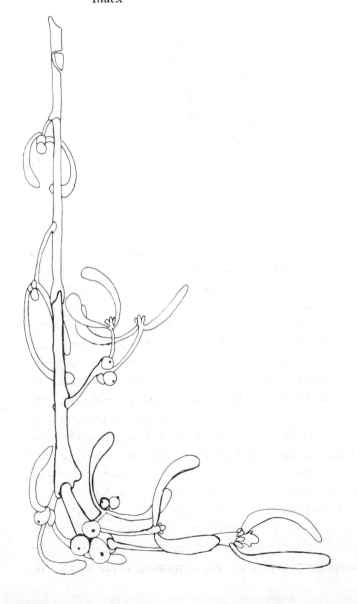

Introduction

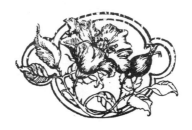

During these last 25 years in which I have been creating recipes and formulas for taking care of myself and my family, many situations have occurred that made us very thankful for this type of information. Even though we live in a large and very sophisticated city it is always beneficial to be able to create some needed item out of the contents of a cabinet or the odds and ends that fill my home's many nooks and crannies. When I purchased a beautiful wool coat and discovered that the price of a moth repellent hangar was $12, I knew that I could make one myself for much less with what I had on hand. When the newly arrived Siberian Husky pup took one look at my never-before-desecrated rugs and immediately defecated, my son suggested that using kitty litter might help. I threw a handful of the litter into the blender, ground it up on low speed, added a few drops of Cedar oil (but Rosemary oil or any other would work as well), and added an equal amount of baking soda. After gathering up the large chunky stuff we spread about a half-inch layer of my "Mess Remover" over the remaining urine and mess.

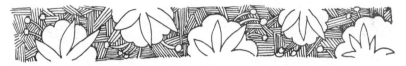

During the next few minutes we could see the liquid coming *up* (rather than going down and into the carpet) as it was absorbed by our mixture, and in about 5 minutes I was able to vacuum up the remaining mess. The result was a stain-free and odor-free carpet. This mixture can also be used for baby vomit or any other noxious substance inadvertently dropped on a carpet. On other occasions and for various reasons I have created scented notepaper, scented ink, scented glue for home and school projects, delicate cleansers for antique woods, and techniques to clean my paintings after they were dirtied by next-door construction projects. It is true that my kids have on occasion said to me, "Mom, you're sort of weird, but everyone always likes to find out what strange thing you are going to invent next."

Recently, when I developed a serious lung condition, I needed to stay away from all known allergens and any substances that were known to cause allergies. Rather than pay for expensive books that would tell me what products I could and could not use, I made them. Laundry detergent was an important item that I needed to make and TSP (trisodium phosphate) and baking soda was the perfect substitute for my usual brand. Eventually, it turned out that I was not allergic to the contents of most detergents. And yet the experiment was well worth it, for the substitute I had learned to make was more effective than the commercial brands in cleaning clothes and left a wonderfully fresh scent. Besides, it cost much less.

As for our health, Jeanne Rose's house is probably one of the few where aspirin and Band-Aids do not have a place on the shelf. My home remedies for common health and sports prob-

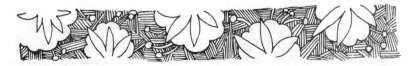

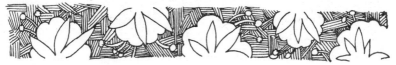

lems are extremely effective, extremely gentle, and very cost effective. My friends appreciate the modernness of my pioneer remedies, especially now that there is so much fear about crazy people poisoning the local pharmacy's stocks and the new studies that have shown that the so-called standard remedies available in stores often do not work at all. Homeopathic and herbal first aid work on both pets and babies, so you can't say these remedies are only successful with patients who regain their health by sheer force of will power. Those old saws, "If you think it works, it probably will," or, "It's just the placebo effect," don't apply. I have seen more babies go quietly off to sleep after a modern mommy, all dressed up to go to work, gave her child a homeopathic tablet of Camomile and held the child for a few minutes before she left.

It *is* difficult for modern mothers, who have to work, to leave their baby in the hands of a sitter. But by leaving a few simple and *harmless* remedies available to the sitter, Mom can go off to work and do her job competently knowing that the baby will be well taken care of. Teenagers are notoriously difficult, emotionally and physically. They literally sprout overnight like Corn in a field. If you have ever been in a cornfield you can indeed see it grow overnight. But some of the remedies listed in this book, such as clay for odor, dry shampoo for oily hair, and some remedies for acne, will go far to improve teenagers' outlook on life.

In our modern life, delicious new ideas about food give us another reason to become reacquainted with the use of the good herbs. And growing these herbs indoors is easy using the few

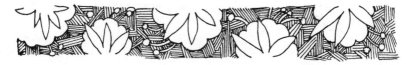

simple ideas in the following pages. I hope that after reading this book it will become clear to you that nothing has only one use. The herbal mixture you used in your bath or as a medicine to give the baby will find use as a fertilizer for your potted plants, or the Roses your husband gave you can be dried and used as potpourri. All herbal ideas have many ramifications and extensions in the herbal *and* modern home. How interesting it is that our modern homes are reliving the creative thinking of our cabin past.

I have written an entire book, *Jeanne Rose's Herbal Body Book,* on the use of herbs externally for beauty and good looks, but the chapter in this book on dieting is new and will help keep you slim and handsome, while the chapter on beauty products contains my latest ideas and favoritie goodies.

Using the aromatic herbs and scents as therapy may be a rather exotic thought, and though some folks find the ideas new and enchanting, they also are tried and true remedies of our past. Scent and color added to your life will enchant, delight, *and* heal both your spirit and your health.

This book truly is a *Modern Herbal.*

Jeanne Rose
April 1987

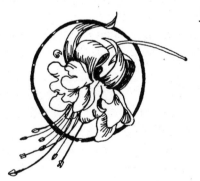

1

· · ·

The Herbal Home

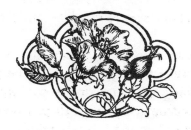

Incense, good herbal smells wafting through the house, natural formulas for cleaning, cleansing, and scenting—this is what I mean when I say "the herbal household." I could also call it the natural household. Why waste your money in the supermarket on expensive commercial household commodities when the same items can so easily be made at home joyfully and inexpensively. In this era of reduced expectations we can live more elegantly and still save money by testing our ingenuity and resources and resorting to the timely, tried-and-true recipes and formulas of our pioneer past.

The kitchen will be covered in Chapter 6. I'll start here with recipes for potpourri, body oil, ink, cleansers, cleaners, laundry scenters, spot removers, making soap from leftover pieces, herbal smokes, incense, insect repellents, and moth-repellent hangers for clothing.

OLD-FASHIONED POTPOURRI
made from store-bought herbs flowers

You probably do not have a garden that yields enough herbs and flowers to make potpourri to scent your house and to give away as gifts. But don't despair—simply order herbs from your favorite mail-order herb store or buy direct and make your own potpourri. When you order, make sure that you get the brightest red and darkest blue flowers so that your potpourri will be really dazzling.

1/2	lb coarse dark brown sugar, sprinkled with 1 oz Rose or Rose Geranium essential oil (or other sweetly scented oil) and ¼ oz Cinnamon oil, and stored in an airtight container for 1 month.
1	bu or 5 lb of brightly colored petals, such as Rose, Poppy, Peony, or Malva, thoroughly mixed and each scented with its own scents.
1	lb Sandalwood pieces that have been sprinkled with Sandalwood oil and stored for a month
3	oz coarse-ground or whole Cloves
3	oz mixed spices, Allspice, Cinnamon, Mace, cut or powdered
2	oz Orris root, cut
1	oz Benzoin or Storax gum, coarsely ground
1	oz Calamus root, cut
1	oz Cinnamon sticks, crushed into large pieces

After the sugar, petals, and Sandalwood have absorbed the scent of the essential oils, mix with the rest of the ingredients. Put the entire 7½ pounds of potpourri in a large garbage sack and store in a dark, dry place for a few weeks so that all the scents will blend. Then you can put the potpourri into attractive containers, stuff fabric bags as drawer scenters, or fill attractive baskets to add drama and scent to your home and to give as gifts.

SOOTHING BODY OIL FOR MASSAGE OR DRY SKIN

Any mixture of oils is helpful for dry and irritated skin, or to add to the pleasures of a massage. But in my experience several mixtures have proven more effective than others. One I favor is made from equal quantities of Corn oil, Olive oil, and Peanut oil. To 8 ounces of this mixture I add 1 ounce Wheat germ oil and ¼ ounce of an essential oil. Sage oil is especially good for sore muscles, and Rose or Orange oil for dry or tense skin; Peppermint oil stimulates; Pennyroyal oil rubbed onto an animal acts as a bug repellent; and Lemongrass oil is a good antidote for oily skin.

SCENTED NOTEPAPER

You will need strongly scented oils and herbs, such as Rosemary, Lemon Verbena, Lemon, or Peppermint. Mix whatever oils you like, or just use one. You will need only 1 ounce of oil. If you like Lemon Verbena, saturate a few pieces of cotton with the oil and wring out. Put a layer of the same herb into the bottom of your stationery box, then the pieces of scented cotton, then a layer of muslin, and finally the paper and envelopes. Keep the box covered. Your paper will eventually become nicely scented with the aroma you have chosen and this will ultimately become your trademark scent.

SCENTED INK

In a tiny, tightly covered pan, simmer together 1 ounce of herb (Lemon Verbena, or whatever, to match your scented paper) and ½ cup of water. The fresher the herb, the more strongly scented it will be. Simmer until the water has almost evaporated. Strain the herb water carefully through a strainer and squeeze all the liquid out of the herbs. To this liquid add a few drops of essential oil compatible with the herb, and mix this together with a 59-milliliter (2-ounce) bottle of ink. I generally use brown ink because the herbal decoction always turns out somewhat brown in color. An alternative method is to mix a few drops of an essential oil with a few drops of alcohol and add this directly to the bottle of ink.

MAKING BLACK INK FROM SCRATCH

A good writing ink should flow readily from the pen, show a good color, and not damage either the pen or the paper. Sediment should not form in the pen, though it is acceptable in the inkstand. It should not be possible to obliterate the ink by water or alcohol. So begins the recipe for ink in the *Techno-Chemical Receipt Book* of 1919. It goes on to give a recipe that is easily made and scented for home use.

12   parts of Gall-nuts, coarsely ground and boiled, or better yet, digested in 120 parts water that is near boiling

Strain and filter the decoction and then add 5 parts sulfate of iron and 5 parts of gum Senegal.

The following is another recipe using more specific measurements: Boil 1 pound of pulverized Gall-nuts in ½ gallon of water, strain the decoction through a linen cloth and filter it, and add ½ pound each of sulfate of iron and gum-Arabic dissolved in 1½ quarts of water. Stir the mixture from time to time and expose it to the air until it has attained a bluish-black color. Then allow it to settle and draw off and bottle the clear ink. To prevent mould from forming in the ink, add 1 drop of Creosote for every quart of ink and stir it in thoroughly.

HOMEMADE CLEANSERS AND CLEANERS

You can make a simple cleaner for all painted surfaces from ammonia, vinegar, and baking soda. I like to use a mixture of ammonia and white vinegar that I have scented with Lemon or Lemon Verbena oil. The formula calls for 1 cup of ammonia, ½ cup white vinegar plus 4 drops Lemon oil, and ¼ cup baking soda. Store this mixture in a glass bottle marked *Wall Cleaner* and include the ingredients on the label. Use ½ cup or more of the basic mixture to every quart of warm to hot water.

Equal parts of mineral oil and mineral spirits will make an excellent mixture for cleaning and polishing natural wood surfaces. You can add Lemon oil to this mixture to nicely scent the polished woods. Store this in a wide-mouthed canning-style jar and label it *Wood Cleaner and Polish*. Polish with a soft cloth after cleaning the wood.

You can make *Scouring Powder for Porcelain* from a substance called whiting, a form of calcium carbonate, available in hardware stores. To 8 ounces of whiting, add 1 ounce of powdered laundry detergent and ½ ounce of finely ground pumice. Mix and store in a well-covered jar that is appropriately labeled. This powder is not suitable for painted walls but works well on porcelain.

You can make a good *Floor Cleaner* from equal quantities of Lemon or Pine-scented ammonia and plain baking soda. Add a cup of this mixture to a gallon or less of hot water and use it to clean kitchen and bathroom floors.

You can make *Laundry Detergent* from TSP (trisodium phosphate) and borax. TSP is available from some hardware stores and costs about $6 for 5 pounds. Compare this price and the quantity needed to do a load of laundry and you will see how economical it is. To every load of laundry, add 2 tablespoons of TSP and ½ cup of Borax. This is a fabulous detergent, better than most that are available commercially. Another advantage is that it can be used by persons with allergies who are affected by commercial products.

LAUNDRY SCENTERS

In the last rinse of your laundry cycle, add ¼ teaspoon essential oil of Lavender dissolved in a bit of alcohol. Another method is to stuff a muslin bag with the herb Lavender and throw this into the last rinse. You can reuse the muslin bag until its scent is gone. It can also be used in your bath as a rubdown for the skin and as a scent for the bathwater.

SPOT REMOVER

For use on natural fabrics, such as cotton, linen, or wool: Grate 1 cup of castile soap into a wide-mouth quart jar and add ½ cup oil of Rosemary and 1 ounce 75 percent alcohol. Mix these ingredients and store them in a hot and sunny place. Eventually the soap will melt and blend with the oil and alcohol. To use, take a small amount, work up into a foam and rub the foam into the spot on both sides of the garment or rug. Try to work up a good foam. Then rinse off the excess or launder the garment. Rosemary oil has a powerful fragrance and can be used as a repellent to animals when spot cleaning rugs. Dilute a few drops of oil with a few tablespoons of water and rub into the cleaned fabric, or add several drops of the oil in the last part of the laundry cycle.

For removing the stain and smell of urine and feces on a rug: As soon as possible after the accident, pour an entire box of baking soda over the spot. Let the baking soda soak up all the liquid and smell. In about 36 to 48 hours the poop can be easily picked up in an entire unpleasant hunk and the area vacuumed. Urine will be absorbed almost entirely. The stain or spot, if there is one, can then be cleaned with the Spot Remover.

MAKING SOAP FROM LEFTOVER PIECES

Start by collecting soap pieces over the course of the year. I have an attractive pottery container for just this purpose in the bathroom. Because I intend to recycle the leftovers I feel no remorse about discarding a piece of soap before it becomes a tiny bit of pulp. My pottery container holds about a pint. When the container is full of soap pieces of all colors and varieties— this takes about 6 months of continual saving in my small family—I grate it coarsely into a small enamel pan. (This produces about 2 cups of soap.) Then I add ½ cup of hot water and let it sit for an hour. When the soap has absorbed the water, I like to add 2 ounces of Rose or Orange flower water. Heat over boiling water (double boiler) for a few minutes to start the soap melting; while it is heating cut with a pastry blender or mix with a wooden spoon. The more you whip it the more likely you will obtain a floating soap. This will leave the soap fairly well blended with bits and pieces of color showing (that is, if you started with colored soap).

When it is fairly well blended I add an essential oil that has been mixed with a solvent such as vegetable oil or alcohol (to about ½ teaspoon of essential oil add 5 teaspoons of either solvent). The solvent is not really essential but the oil does soothe the skin and the alcohol can help to degrease oily skin. You can also mix the essential oil with flower water and add it to the soap. Of course, the flower water and the essential oil are only an aesthetic improvement.

Now, all you have to do is roll the soap up into balls or press it into a mold of some sort. I have used coddled egg cups, poached egg cups, small cream jars, and other cup-shaped objects to press my soap in. After the soap is pressed into the mold, let it sit for a few weeks to dry and harden. Then it is ready for use.

WINTER INCENSE

Mix 1 ounce each of Lavender, Cloves, Orris root, Benzoin gum, and Cinnamon. The Lavender can be in bud form but the rest should be coarsely ground or powdered. Mix 1 teaspoon each of oil of Lemon, oil of Clove, oil of Lavender, and oil of Cinnamon. Mix the liquid with the powdered herbs and store in an airtight, lightproof container until needed. When needed, stir the contents and put a small amount into a metal dish or ashtray. Place this on top of a heater. The heat activates the scent and vaporizes the volatile oil into the air, where it will aromatize your house with a delicate, warming scent.

HERBAL SMOKES

There are a number of herbs that are smoked, both for their medicinal purposes and for pleasure. If you roll your own cigarettes as I once did, you can add anything you like to the tobacco to gain whatever benefits you desire. I rolled pure Virginia leaf—I believe the brand was called Three Castles—into delicately flavored cigarettes. I smoked Tobacco for 18 years before I was able to give up this disgusting habit. Although there are a few herbal smokes that have medicinal effects, I would strongly recommend that you avoid smoking altogether, whether it be Tobacco or herbs. There is nothing wholesome about smoking; very occasionally, however, herbs will give results when smoked that no tea or infusion can duplicate.

If you want to stop smoking Tobacco and are puffing on herbs to escape the dread nicotine habit, you are limited to just a few herbal smokes. Pipe smokers are always benefiting from herbs, since most pipe Tobaccos are cured with various herbs to improve the taste, smell, and quality of the smoke. Crushed, Allspice adds fragrance to Tobacco. Bearberry leaves make cigarettes milder. Comfrey, added to the pipe or the cigarette, has a healing effect on the lungs. Deer Tongue and Licorice flavor Tobacco, Rosemary and Sage are smoked by themselves to dry mucus and excess secretions from the lungs. Yerba Santa has an aromatic scent and flavor when smoked; when chewed it is first bitter and resinous, then cooling and sweet. Yerba Santa is especially healing to the lungs and is good mixed with Sage. Smoking Marjoram, Camomile, and Gentian is said to help cure Tobacco habit. This mixture can also be drunk as a tea to help the addicted become unaddicted. A spicy blend of herbs called "David Copperfield," made of Mullein, Cubeb, and Lobelia, is said to help those who wish to quit smoking. Asthmatics can take a puff or two of Datura to ease their asthmatic sufferings.

INSECT REPELLENTS

Insect repellents can be made from almost any strongly aromatic essential oil or herb. The best herbs, however, are Mugwort, Wormwood, Pennyroyal, Bay, Eucalyptus, Lavender, Rose Geranium, and Thyme. The herbs and essential oils can be used singly or in combinations. To make a house fragrant for guests put a drop of Rose oil on some of the light bulbs, especially those near the door. To deter flying insects substitute insect-repelling oils such as Thyme or Lavender. For creeping insects, dilute Thyme, Lavender, Pennyroyal, and Bay oils with alcohol and use a toothbrush or tiny paintbrush to paint all cracks, crevices, corners, and baseboards with it. The formula can also be used under rugs.

Pennyroyal herb is especially good for flea control, while Bay leaves are better for tiny beetles. A useful insect repellent for bags, drawers, hangers, suitcases, and trunks is made with the herbs Mugwort, Sage, or Santolina with Thyme oil added.

INSECT REPELLENT RECIPE

1   cup each of Mugwort, Santolina, Sage, Rose Geranium, and Lavender
1   tsp Thyme oil dropped onto and mixed with ½ cup salt
1   handful each of Bay leaves and Cloves

Mix everything and use as directed.

MOTH-REPELLENT HANGERS
for Fine Woolens, Pants, Coats

For 4 hangers you will need 4 sturdy wooden hangers, 1–2 pounds of Herbal Moth Repellent, and 4 pieces of nice cotton cloth 8 inches by 13 inches. The herbal mixture can be made of equal quantities of Pennyroyal herb, Camomile flowers, and Spearmint; Bay leaves mixed with Eucalyptus leaves; or simply Cedar shavings that you have picked up at the lumberyard. For this mixture it's best to use whole, dried leaves and flowers or ones that are coarsely cut. 1) Curl the fabric into a 13-inch-long tube over the lower edge of the hanger and sew a seam into this long edge. 2) Take a piece of string or pretty ribbon and tightly tie to close off one end of the tube. 3) Stuff the open end of the tube with the herbal mixture. It will take at least 4 ounces of herbs. 4) Tie the open end tightly to contain the herbs.

The scent and repellent properties of the herbs will seep through the cloth to whatever is on the hanger, keeping it safe from moths and bugs. In a year or so it will be an easy matter to refresh your herbal mixture by untying one end of the cloth tube and replacing the herbs with a fresh mixture.

2

. . .

Herbal Home Remedies

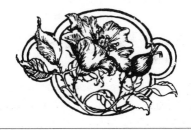

- Athlete's Foot
- Bee Stings or Insect Bites
- Blisters
- Bowel and Stomach Distress
- Bruises
- Burns
- Coldness or Frostbite
- Colds and Fevers
- Crotch Rash or Diaper Rash
- Crushed Fingers and Toes
- Cuts and Scratches
- Earaches
- Eyes—Irritated, Sore or Tired

- Fever (see Colds)
- Headache
- Insomnia
- Jet Lag
- Nosebleed
- Poisoning
- Poison Oak or Ivy
- Sore Muscles
- Sprains
- Stomachache (see Bowel and Stomach Distress)
- Sunburn
- Sunstroke or Heatstroke
- Toothache
- Vomiting and Flatulence

Home remedies for common illnesses have much to do with herbal medicine. And herbal medicine is intimately associated with the history of mankind. The origin of many simple home medicines dates from prehistory, a time before records were kept. Certainly early man looked to the animals and observed how diligently they searched out certain plants when a health crisis of any kind occurred. And man certainly followed their lead—was not man at that time very close to an animal himself? Over eons of time, through the observation of healing techniques and the trial-and-error process of their application, man learned how to care for his medical needs. This and a simple, wholesome diet of fresh fruits and vegetables, some meat, and regular exercise kept our ancestors in good physical health.

Eventually the "magic" of this simple healing using plants and herbs became the responsibility of the priest or learned physician. Man slowly gave up the responsibility for his physical care to such "experts." But the country people always maintained some storehouse of this knowledge and continued to care for themselves and their domestic animals.

Accurate information about medicinal plants and their properties and applications is found in several ancient manuscripts. The Ebers Papyrus, which dates from 1500 B.C., and the *Nei Ching,* a Chinese medical work that dates from 2500 B.C., are two of the oldest and most authoritative sources. The information from these works was later transcribed in several other ancient Chinese and Greek works. And herbals continued to be written from that time to the present. During the early part of this century here in the United States, called the era of "modern

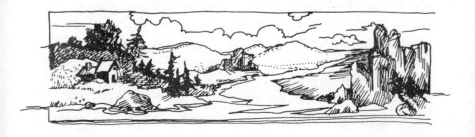

medicine," certain fantastic discoveries relating to germs and synthesized medicines were made. Aspirin, or its native derivative, was isolated from a bark that had been originally gathered by herbal collectors from the species of Willow tree called *Salix alba*. This knowledge was gained from wise American Indians. The substance was synthesized, processed, and sold as tablets rather than pieces of bark.

Now, how many people know that one of our most commonly used medicines, aspirin, was originally a bark tea drunk for aches and pains? Digitalis is extracted from Foxglove, morphine from Poppy; quinine, now replaced by synthetic drugs, comes from a Peruvian tree. Colchicine, used for gout, is derived from the autumn Crocus, and penicillin is derived from penicillium, a mold that also makes a delicious blue cheese. These and many, many other plants are examples of how we have used traditional plant wisdom to heal ourselves.

But what about our own modern age with its unique health hazards: the pollution that endangers our respiratory system, pesticides and poisons on our foods, impure water with asbestos particles? Can we still use simple plants to heal or will we always have to go to medical doctors? Professional medical care comes at a dreadful cost of time, energy, and money, and most often we are simply told to go home and rest, because whatever it is will go away eventually. Maybe we're also given an expensive chemical medicine to counteract the chemical illness that we have contracted.

Herbal medicine is home medicine. Herbal medicine is simple medicine, harmless, gentle, easy to use, with very few side effects. How much better it would be to gain a repertoire of knowledge about a few common substances that one could use to treat most of the common ailments that we encounter daily.

The herbal revolution is now; we are a part of the herbal renaissance. A rebirth of our native wisdom is occurring, partly from the example of the Chinese and other cultures that have continued to use plants for health from the beginning.

Herbs heal, sometimes slowly and sometimes imperceptibly,

but they do heal. Herbal teas and tinctures taken regularly will often cure even the most persistant ailment. But herbs and simple remedies show the most dramatic results in the everyday problems that beset us: the blisters, insect bites, rashes, colds, earaches, and bowel troubles that are common occurrences. These are what we will deal with in this section, and with common, safe herbs and things that are easy to use and economical.

HOME REMEDIES FOR SIMPLE AILMENTS

Athlete's Foot.This fungus infection results when the chemical balance of the foot changes due to environmental changes such as increased moisture or heat. The toes should be kept clean, washed, and dry. White socks that can be sterilized by boiling should be worn. The feet can be washed with soap and then rinsed or soaked in Apple cider vinegar or honey water twice a day. Before putting on your socks, sprinkle the area between the toes with a mixture of Golden Seal and clay. The clay absorbs the moisture while the Golden Seal helps to destroy the fungus.

HEALING DUSTING POWDER

Mix 1 part Golden Seal powder and 1 part cosmetic clay, bottle, label, and use wherever there is a problem with moisture or a rash. This mixture can be used for athlete's foot, diaper rash, or crotch itch.

Bee Stings or Insect Bites. As soon as a bee stings or a bug bites, remove the stinger of the bee and rub the area vigorously with any green herb handy. This releases chlorophyll, which has a quick soothing and pain-killing action on the sting. The best herbs to use are Savory, Plantain, or Comfrey, but even grass will do in a pinch. A moistened tea bag is also useful as a poultice. My preference would be either Papaya leaf tea or any black tea. The healing dusting powder mentioned above is very soothing and can be used after the initial "sting" goes away. If you have bottled chlorophyll, this can be dabbed on the irritation whenever necessary. Another useful remedy is a paste of Chlorella and water. Chlorella has a chlorophyll content of 75 percent, the highest in the plant world. Chlorella can also be taken by mouth to detoxify the body in case there is an allergic reaction to the bee sting or insect bite. It would probably also be wise to take some pantothenic acid and vitamin C if there is a history of allergy. Straight honey is also excellent as an application for any sting or bite.

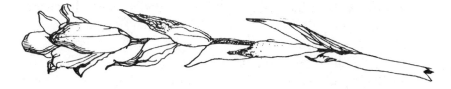

Blisters. My favorite and what I feel is the most effective treatment for blisters is DMSO. DMSO has received FDA approval for use with certain animals, but as not yet received approval for human use. DMSO, dimethyl sulfoxide, is a by-product of the lumber industry and the paper manufacturing process. It is a solvent that has the unique ability to dissolve more chemicals than any other solvent. And it can penetrate the skin, carrying many dissolved chemicals with it and into the bloodstream in seconds. It also freezes a few degrees below room temperature. These properties are also what make it very controversial even though it has been shown to control and cure some diseases. It is possible that if it is applied with dirty hands or dirty tools, harmful substances could be absorbed into the bloodstream. (Read *The Persecuted Drug: The Story of DMSO,* by Pat McGrady, Sr., for a positive account of DMSO; for the negative side of the story ask an informed doctor.)

As soon as I know a blister exists, I apply a bit of DMSO on it, cover with moleskin and leave alone. I realize that many people do not have this substance easily available. The next best thing to do when you find a blister is to make sure it is clean, cover it with moleskin or lamb's wool, and leave it alone. If you must reduce its size, you can sterilize a needle and pierce it where the bubble joins the skin and then cover with a sterile Band-Aid, although again moleskin or lamb's wool provides a nice soft fat cover to the sore spot.

I have used a clay and Golden Seal poultice on my son when he picked up a hot plate and a huge blister formed on the palm of his hand. We put a thick, soft blob of white clay mixed with a bit of Golden Seal on the blister, covered it, and wrapped a towel around his hand. Several hours later, when the clay had dried, my son removed the towel, and found the blister was reduced to the size of a flat quarter, which we covered with a Band-Aid. I have found that Band-Aids by themselves are next to useless on blisters and prefer moleskin or lamb's wool, and would certainly recommend that you always carry one of these in your first aid kit, plus a bit of adhesive to attach it to the skin.

Bowel and Stomach Distress can result from eating too much food, too little food, the wrong combination of foods, unripe or spoiled foods, or strange exotic foods; or trouble may be caused simply by the lack of digestive juices in the body, or be a part of another illness that you are experiencing, or result from stress or tension. If this last is the case it is best to stay away from solid foods altogether until you and your body are calm and relaxed. Bowel or stomach distress can lead to constipation, diarrhea, or dysentery. These are the most common problems, and yet people suffer from them needlessly when simple home remedies can almost immediately rectify the situation. Aloe vera gel is a basic remedy for each of these conditions, and can also be taken for stomachache or ulcers, or used externally on burns.

CONSTIPATION REMEDIES

Constipation may be the result of lifelong improper diet, and this cannot be dealt with in this little paragraph. But if temporary constipation is your problem, try drinking plenty of water or Prune juice to hydrate the bowel, or eat Bran flakes to provide bulk. At night drink ½ cup of Olive oil in ½ cup of Orange juice. Lighten your food load with simple steamed vegetables until the bowels move. You may also need to take an Olive oil enema to break up the hard bulk so that it can pass. My favorite commercial product, which also finds use as a face-steaming mixture, is Swiss Kriss, a combination of herbs that includes Licorice and Senna leaf. If you prefer a single herbal remedy, then take Senna pod tea. It is less griping than Senna leaf, that is, it is easier on the system. For a child or old person, 3 to 6 pods are steeped in 1 cup of cool water, and then the liquid is drunk; for an adult, take 6 to 12 pods, steeped in cold water, strained and drunk.

STOMACHACHE/DIARRHEA/ DYSENTERY REMEDIES

Do you remember the activated charcoal that you put into your fish tank to adsorb gases and odors and clean the water? You can use the same thing for stomach or intestinal distress. The charcoal is processed from pure vegetable ingredients and can adsorb many, many times its weight in irritating gases and toxins. It also combats bad odor and reduces cramps. For a stomachache, diarrhea, or dysentery take 2 to 3 of these charcoal tablets and drink a cup or two of Papaya leaf tea. This is the best remedy, but if you have neither of these then 1 to 2 teaspoons of liquid chlorophyll will also do the job. But activated charcoal, like moleskin, is simple and cheap and should be kept in everyone's home. Activated charcoal never enters the bloodstream but works entirely in the digestive tract. It has a highly porous surface, which is able to adsorb tremendous amounts of gas and toxins. This is truly a "simple," that is, a single remedy used to treat a particular condition. It has been in use for at least 2,000 years to treat gas and diarrhea.

Bruises. A bruise is caused by a blow or compression that leaves the skin unbroken but breaks small blood vessels beneath the surface, which causes soreness and discoloration. Bruises are best treated by the instant application of cold water or ice wrapped in a cloth. A homeopathic remedy called Arnica tincture, or Bellis perennis tincture, or the herbal remedy called Calendula oil, are excellent when applied. A gentle application of any of these can be very effective. Taking a sufficient quantity of vitamin C and bioflavenoids encourages the basic integrity of the tissues and bruising will not be nearly as severe or painful.

Burns. Aloe vera gel, honey, or simple vitamin E are the easiest and most effective remedies for a burn. An Aloe vera plant grown in the kitchen is useful and handy, and if you get burned, just cut a bit of leaf and apply the cool gel from the inside of the leaf to the burn. Honey, most effective to cool and heal a burn, is usually handy and can be instantly applied forming a protective cover that allows the burn to heal very quickly.

Coldness or Frostbite. Warm the area by immersing in body-temperature water or by pressing the cold area next to a warm person. Frostbite has also been successfully treated by direct applications of DMSO. Cold hands or feet can be warmed by sprinkling Cayenne pepper into the socks before putting them on, or on the palms of the hands, which are then rubbed together. Remember, do not put your hands in your eyes! (If this happens the eyes will burn and hurt but no permanent damage will occur. Cayenne pepper in the eyes can be treated by a direct application of yogurt.) Coldness can also be treated by warming a bit of Olive oil and adding a few drops of Rosemary oil for every ounce of Olive oil. This is then rubbed onto the cold area, first gently, then more vigorously, until you are using friction (called a friction rub). A half-teaspoon of Cayenne can also be taken in ½ glass of water every 2 hours to warm you from the inside out—this improves circulation. Another favorite method of mine is to simmer a 1-inch-square sliced piece of Ginger in a cup of water for 10 minutes, adding a few grains of Cayenne and maybe a bouillon cube, and then to drink this soup. This is most healthy and very warming.

Colds and Fevers. At the first sign of a cold take plenty of vitamin C, reduce the complexity of the foods you are eating to just a few simple choices, wrap a nice woolly scarf around your neck and slow down your life a bit. If you have a fever, run a vaporizer in your house with a few drops of Peppermint oil in the well to "cool" you, or if chills are the problem add Cinnamon oil, Rosemary oil or Basil oil to the vaporizer to "warm" you. Respiratory congestion calls for Eucalyptus oil.

Keep a supply of Garlic oil perles in the house. These come in mighty handy either as an application to insect bites, to squeeze into an aching ear, to take internally if you have stomach distress, or to "kill" the virus that is causing the cold. Take 3 Garlic perles every 4 hours, plus ½ teaspoon Cayenne, plus some vitamin C tablets, about 1 gram per hour.

With a really serious cold or fever it is a good idea to strengthen the lymphatic system with a mixture of herbs noted for their cleansing and blood-purifying abilities.

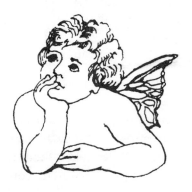

BLOOD PURIFIER FOR COLDS

2   oz Echinacea root—helps the body build its own resistance and increase the number of leukocytes, which counteract infection

1   oz Yellow Dock root—a noted blood purifier

1   oz Golden Seal root—has powerful antibacterial action

1/2   oz Ginseng root—encourages and stimulates all the organ systems

These herbs (roots) are purchased in powdered form, mixed, and stuffed into gelatin capsules, size 00 (double naught). Two capsules are taken 3 times per day for not more than 10 days.

These simple treatments will ease any discomfort you may have and may totally eliminate any illness whatsoever.

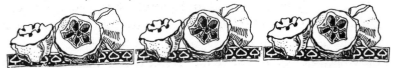

Crotch Rash or Diaper Rash. This can be caused by any number of situations from too acid skin or secretions to too alkaline ones. The area should be kept clean and dry by washing with a gentle, neutral soap and plain water and powdering with clay. Honey, yogurt, and lecithin are also excellent applications for a rash of any kind. If the rash is particularly irritating, use a mixture of 4 teaspoons clay and 1 teaspoon each, in powdered form, of vitamin C and Golden Seal root. If a wet discharge is also part of the rash, add 1 teaspoon of powdered Comfrey root, which will prove very healing.

Crushed Fingers and Toes. These are best treated by soaking as long as you possibly can in an infusion of Comfrey root. Comfrey is healing and helps to soothe the pain. If you have it, take 4 drops tincture of Arnica in ½ cup water every 15 minutes or so. Arnica tincture or Calendula oil can also be applied externally.

Cuts and Scratches. Wash carefully with soap. This is all that is necessary for a small cut. A large cut or deep scratch can be washed with a weak tea of Golden Seal or Echinacea root. Large cuts may also need to be closed with a butterfly Band-Aid. Even deep cuts that may look like they need stitches can be taken care of at home.

Once while cutting Garlic, I sliced the end off my finger, including part of the fingernail. I could not find the piece of finger in the Garlic so had to content myself with stanching the flow of blood and easing the pain. I tried to apply a chewed-up piece of Comfrey leaf, which only made the raw end hurt more. Fortunately I keep an infusion of Comfrey root and Fennel seed in the refrigerator for stomachache and as an eyewash. So I stuck my whole finger into the cold bottle of Comfrey/Fennel tea and left it there for about an hour. Then I soaked a very soft piece of cloth in the liquid and loosely wrapped my finger overnight. By the next morning granular healing tissue was forming, and within days the finger was healed.

If you do not get to your cut or scratch in time and it becomes infected, you should soak it in a very hot cleansing solution, such as soap and water. The hot Comfrey/Fennel eyewash would also work, as would plain hot water and salt. When the wound is open and draining, apply a poultice of clay. When the clay poultice is totally dry, remove it, rinse the area, and dust with Golden Seal.

Earache. I cannot think of anything more painful than an earache. Pity the poor baby howling with pain from a painful ear—and what is the mother to do? Warmth, love, and your healing hands can often be the whole cure for an earache, but warm Olive oil slid down the external ear canal is very soothing. I especially recommend Garlic oil perles. Pierce one with a needle and squeeze the contents into each ear, even the one that is unaffected. If it is a child with the earache, hold a hot water bottle to the painful ear or hold the child against your body and rock in a rocking chair until the child sleeps.

The earache may be caused by impacted or solid earwax. If this is the case a warm Comfrey infusion can be used as an earwash. You should use an ear syringe and Comfrey water as warm as possible. Suck up the strained Comfrey water into the ear syringe and squeeze the liquid into the affected ear. To determine the proper pressure, first try it out on yourself. Never, never do anything to a child that you have not already tried on yourself. Continue to wash out the ear until the pieces of wax come out with the liquid. Then fill the ear with warm Olive oil, Garlic oil, or Mullein flower oil and plug with a bit of cotton. Some people have hard earwax, and they may have to wash out their ears regularly for their entire lives.

One woman that I met, thinking that Garlic oil meant pure, undiluted oil, used the extracted concentrate as an ear oil. This concentrated substance ate totally through the eardrum, which had to be repaired surgically. When we talk about Garlic oil perles we mean Garlic oil that has been diluted with vegetable oil and is sold in little gelatin capsules. These are sold in health food shops. For first aid you should purchase only this infused Garlic oil, and please read the label.

Exhaustion. The best remedy for exhaustion is rest. Drink a cup of tea, any kind of noncaffeinated tea, and take a nap. However, if for some reason you must continue working or driving, there are a number of herbs that are quite stimulating. Guarana or Yerba maté with their high content of caffeine can be drunk as a tea or taken in capsule form.

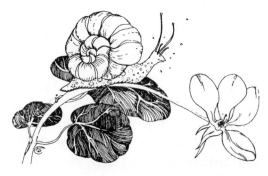

HERBAL STIMULANT

Mix equal quantities of Guarana, Yerba maté, Echinacea, Ginseng, and Rosemary. Brew a tea in the regular way and drink 1 or 2 cups at a time.

HERBAL STIMULANT CAPSULES

Take the above mixture, grind in a seed mill or coffee grinder, and stuff into gelatin capsules. Take 2 capsules (00) every 2–4 hours. Take the tea or capsules as needed but do not use frequently.

Eyes—Irritated, Sore, or Tired. Watching television, reading in poor light, exhaustion, smoky rooms, and air pollution are a few of the reasons why your poor eyes might get sore and red. My only remedy is a cool solution of Fennel seeds and Comfrey root (see p. 178 for recipe). If they are particularly irritated you can add Golden Seal, and if they are only a bit sore, honey diluted in water is very effective. To use, simply fill an eyecup or the palm of your hand with the liquid, pour into the eye, and rinse several times. Use this every 2 to 4 hours until the condition is relieved. The Fennel/Comfrey remedy may be used hot, warm, or cold.

VERY GENTLE EYEWASH

Mix 1 teaspoon honey in ¼ cup hot water. Stir until the honey is dissolved. Use as directed above.

EXTRA-STRONG EYEWASH

To the above formula add 1 teaspoon Golden Seal powder and proceed as directed above.

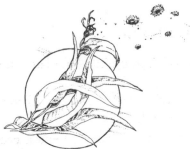 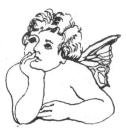

Headache. Rub your temples with a bit of Rosemary oil; do 5 minutes of vigorous calisthenics; put a cool compress of Apple cider vinegar on your forehead; drink a cup of Rosemary or Valerian tea. If the headache is accompanied by a stomachache drink a cup of Camomile tea. A cup of Cabbage soup is also an old folk remedy for headache, as is a compress of Cabbage leaves on the forehead.

Headaches can be caused by certain chemicals, alcohol, even bright light or sunlight. These are trigger situations that should be avoided by those prone to headaches. Some wines have substances that trigger a headache in a susceptible person. Another chemical trigger is the nitrite/nitrate group, which is used as a preservative in salami, hot dogs, processed foods, and canned foods. Chocolate and Coffee can also trigger a headache. This is just another reason why foods like these should be avoided generally. Simple foods like vegetables, fruits, and grains are much better for you.

Insomnia. If for some reason you are unable to sleep, get up. Do some work, exercise vigorously for 10 minutes, take out a difficult book and begin to read. These simple remedies should put anyone to sleep. The very act of brewing a pot of tea is time-consuming, relaxing, and sleep-inducing. Camomile, Valerian, Birch leaves, Lemon Verbena, and Red clover are all sleep-inducing herbs, and a pot of tea made from one of these will ease you into the world of sleep. These herbs can be used individually or in combination. Just use whatever you have. If you are fortunate and have a good herbal repertoire at hand your tea could be:

SLEEP TEA

Formula 1:	1 part each of Camomile, Valerian, and Mint
Formula 2:	1 part each of Lemon verbena, Birch leaves, and Red Clover
Formula 3:	1 part each of Lemon Verbena, Lemon peel, and Valerian

Brew these teas in the usual way, that is, 1 tablespoon of mixed herbs to every cup of boiling water. Let steep for about 3 to 5 minutes, strain, add honey if desired, drink slowly.

My mother's favorite sleep remedy was a barely warm glass of milk to which she added 1 teaspoon of honey and a drop of Vanilla. This never failed to put her to sleep. I use this remedy for my son, who is one of those creatures who just hates for the day to end. He drinks his warm honeyed milk while I read, and more often than not he is asleep within 30 minutes.

Jet Lag. Put a few drops of Rosemary oil in ½ cup of water and drink. In a few hours or at normal bedtime drink a cup of Valerian tea.

Nosebleed. If your nose starts bleeding, lie down, pinch the nostrils shut with two fingers, and keep shut for at least 15 minutes or until your nose stops bleeding. A Rosemary tea compress on the forehead is also very helpful.

Poisoning. If you have Ipecac (which is a remedy available in a drug store) in the house, follow the directions on the package while you are calling the doctor. Some poisons work very slowly, and if poison is even a bit suspected as causing an illness then by all means go immediately to a doctor and follow his directions. If the poisoning is in the form of a sick stomach or grumbling bowels, take charcoal tablets. Every house should have a chart, easily accessible, that lists various poisons and how to treat them, but with our infinite array of chemicals, cleansers, and combinations of ingredients, it is often extremely difficult to know what a suspected poison contains. Take charcoal tablets and call the doctor.

Poison Oak or Ivy. Immediately after being exposed to Poison Oak or Ivy, wash the area with a cleansing soap and cool water. Hot water will spread the irritating oil, while cool water contains it. Take plenty of vitamin C and possibly pantothenic acid to contain the "allergic" reaction. Try not to scratch the blisters. Apply or powder the blisters with clay to keep them from itching. Golden Seal is also helpful, although it stains clothing and makes your skin yellow. Chlorophyll liquid is also very helpful to apply to itchy Poison Oak. And of course don't forget a dab of honey. The honey is sticky but whenever you can use it, do, as it is very effective. If the Poison Oak or Ivy is on the legs apply honey or lecithin or both and cover with a cotton sock.

Sore Muscles. When you overexert in exercise or work, your muscles can get sore and tired. Muscles get sore through a buildup of lactic acid that is incompletely metabolized in the muscular tissue. Saffron tea can help. Since Saffron is prohibitively expensive to drink as a tea (one cup would cost about $2), a simple remedy for sore muscles is to massage them and gently exercise until they feel better. A massage with Rosemary oil is even more helpful. One-quarter ounce oil of Rosemary mixed with 8 ounces Olive oil makes a very effective massage oil. Substitute Mint oil if you want stimulation. Relaxing teas are also helpful to ease tension that sore muscles may create.

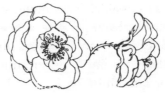

RELAXING TEA

Mix 1 part each Alfalfa, Camomile, Comfrey, Dandelion, Horsetail, and Oatstraw, bottle and label. To use steep one tablespoon of the mixed herbs in 1 cup of hot water for 3 to 5 minutes, strain, and add honey. This is a useful mixture for relaxing and rebuilding worn-out tissues.

Sprains. A sprain is a tear or very marked stretching of a muscle, ligament, or joint. Sprains are very painful and should be treated as soon as possible. Immediate application of cold is helpful, then later, apply heat to relax. Alternate hot and cold soaks are also good for healing the torn tissues. Hot and cold soaks are more helpful when they contain stimulating and relaxing herbs to help in the healing process. They should be done in sequences of 5 minutes hot and 2 minutes cold for at least 20 minutes. A relaxing tea can also be helpful. If you have DMSO, immediately apply it to the sprain and rub it in. Rosemary massage oil is also very useful as a rub.

HOT SOAK FOR SPRAINED OR ACHING MUSCLES OR JOINTS

1   oz Rosemary
1   oz Comfrey root
1   gallon water

Bring the ingredients to a boil in a large flat pan. Turn off the heat and let steep until cool enough to use. The hot soak should be used as hot as possible. This liquid can also be used as a compress and the herbs applied as a plaster. When you can, insert the sprained ankle or hand or sore muscle in the hot water and soak for at least 5 minutes. Then immediately plunge into the cold soak for 2 minutes.

COLD SOAK FOR SPRAINED OR ACHING MUSCLES OR JOINTS

1/4   oz essential oil of Peppermint
1   gallon cold water
2   trays ice cubes

Put all this into a large flat pan. This can be kept for an indefinite period and used whenever necessary as a cold soak for aching muscles or joints. Refrigerate when not in use.

Sunburn. A sunburn is a painful experience. The skin is actually cooked and will eventually peel off to expose fresh new skin underneath. It is, of course, best never to get a sunburn. If your skin is very sensitive, alcohol-based PABA solutions are very helpful to exclude the harmful rays of the sun. Once you get the sunburn, the first thing you must do is to cool the skin. Immersing in a cool bath is good. Adding baking soda to the bath water is even more effective. Vitamin E oil and Aloe Vera gel are noted for their effectiveness in healing a sunburn and should be immediately applied, either one or the other, or alternating them. A cold Comfrey root compress is excellent, and if you have kept the Fennel seed/Comfrey root eyewash made up and in the refrigerator this can be immediately applied to cool and cure a sunburn. Keep reapplying any of these substances until the redness has turned brown and no longer hurts.

Sunstroke or Heatstroke. When your body is simply unable to get rid of excessive heat and your internal temperature goes up too far, sunstroke results. The temperature may climb to 106 to 108 degrees. You may get weak and giddy, feel nauseous, and sweat profusely. The very best thing to do is to submerge your entire body in cool water. A cold cloth on the head or an Apple cider vinegar compress pressed against any part of the body that feels excessively hot will help too. A drop or two of Peppermint oil in a quart of water is very cooling when used as a compress. Also drink plenty of cool (not cold) fluids. Slightly salted water (¼ teaspoon salt per 2 cups of water) is beneficial. Physicians recommend a .1 percent saline solution. You can drink Gatorade or other commercial products that approximate the electrolyte concentration of sweat. Keep cool, but not chilled, rest, and reduce activity during extremely hot spells.

Toothache. Toothaches should no doubt be treated by a competent dentist. But if you cannot get to one quickly enough, a drop of clove oil on a tiny piece of cotton that is then put into or on the aching tooth will quickly ease the pain. Taking bone meal or dolomite tablets is very relaxing and will also help by "feeding" the nerves. The Blood Purifier recipe (given in the Colds and Fevers section above) should also be taken. Sometimes taking these capsules as well as bone meal will cure whatever problem is causing the aching teeth. It should most certainly be tried. I also recommend that you take Garlic oil perles, 2 to 3 every 4 hours until the pain is relieved. Homeopathic pharmacies produce a remedy called Chamomilla, which is in tablet or grain form. It is extremely useful for pain, insomnia, tension, stress, undue anxiety, hyperactivity, and headache. These tablets are very economical and can be taken for any of these conditions (2 to 3 is the proper dose).

Vomiting and Flatulence. Measures and remedies used for stomachache or diarrhea should also be used for vomiting and flatulence. Vomiting induced by a poison should be handled by a physician. If you have traveler's diarrhea, however, or queasiness from traveling with attendant vomiting and odorous flatulence, a very simple remedy is 2 drops of Peppermint oil on a sugar cube, which can be sucked, or 2 drops in ½ glass water. This will stop vomiting and will deodorize your excretions. Sometimes the vomiting must be stopped before the other remedies can be used.

Once in Mexico I woke up in the middle of the night, very flatulent, with dreadful abdominal cramps. I was also vomiting and had diarrhea. What a situation! I sipped a glass of water with Peppermint oil while sitting uncomfortably on the toilet; soon the vomiting eased and I was able to take 3 charcoal tablets with a cup of Papaya tea for the gas and diarrhea. I can't say that I was instantly cured, but I can say that I was able to sleep the night. The fever and chills were relieved the next day with Garlic oil capsules and Cayenne taken in water. I continued sipping the Peppermint water and drank only Papaya leaf tea. Within 3 days all my symptoms and aches and pains were gone, which was not the case with my companion, who refused to take these simple remedies and had continuous diarrhea and fever for 6 long days.

A WAY WITH HERBS

We have mentioned various procedures for using herbs, such as fomentation, infusion, poultice and tincture. Here's a quick rundown of these important terms to clear up any lingering confusion.

Fomentation is a hot and wet poultice used on irritated or inflamed areas.

Infusion is a mixture of herb and water, brought to a boil, removed from the fire, steeped or infused, and used as a drink or an external wash. The proportion is generally 1 ounce herb to 16–20 ounces of water.

Poultice is an application of hot, moist herb or infusion directly to the skin to stimulate circulation or heal an inflamed area.

Tincture is the strained solution of herbs and alcohol to be used internally or externally.

CHART OF SIMPLE HOME REMEDIES AND THEIR APPLICATIONS

Complaint	Plant	Form of Application	Dose	Additional Information
ARTHRITIS AND RHEUMATISM	Alfalfa	Tea		
		Capsules	1–2/day	Contains plant estrogens
	Birch bark	Tea		Use with other herbs
		Compress		Apply when necessary
	Red Clover	Tea		
		Capsules	1–2/day	
	Comfrey leaf or root	Infusion		
		Capsules	2–3/day	
		Compress		Apply when necessary
		Bath	1 oz/bath	
	Devil's Claw	Infusion		Should be soaked overnight
		Tincture	10 drops twice/day	

Complaint	Plant	Form of Application	Dose	Additional Information
ARTHRITIS AND RHEUMATISM	Fenugreek seeds	Infusion		Use all the herb teas together. 1–2 cups/day. ½ oz of mixed herbs/day.
	Rooibos	Tea		
	Rosemary	Tea		
BRONCHITIS	Lavender oil	Inhalation	2 drops each time	Use an aromatic diffuser with pure oils.
	Sandalwood oil	Inhalation	2 drops each time	
	Eucalyptus oil	Inhalation	2 drops each time	
	Coltsfoot	Infusion	1–2 cups/day	
	Thyme	Tea	1 tsp/cup/day	
		Bath	1 T/bath	
		Compress	simple infusion	
	Eucalyptus	Tea	2 leaves/cup	
		Bath	½ oz/bath	
		Compress		
	Golden Seal	Capsules	2 twice/day	do not use more than 10 days

	Herb	Form	Amount	Notes
	Sage	Infusion Bath Compress		use with Cayenne and Thyme
	Cayenne	Tea Capsules Compress	¼ tsp/cup water 2–4 at a time ¼ tsp in water	
BURNS	Comfrey	Compress Gel or salve		
	Aloe	Compress Gel or salve		
COLDS	Licorice	Tea	3 cups hot each day	
	Elder flowers	Infusion Bath Compress	3 cups hot each day	
	Peppermint or Cinnamon	Inhalation	½ T in vaporizer twice/day	
		Infusion Bath Compress		depends on whether there are chills or fever

Complaint	Plant	Form of Application	Dose	Additional Information
COLDS	Basil and Eucalyptus oils	Inhalation	2 drops each time for a 'cold' cold	Use Aroma-Vera diffusor
	Peppermint and Eucalyptus oils	Inhalation	2 drops each time for a 'hot' cold	Use in a diffusion
	Garlic and Cayenne	Capsules	6/day	
CONSTIPATION	Senna pods	Tea	1 cup of 3 pods	
		Capsules	2 oz/day	
		Enema	3 pods plus 1 qt water	
	Olive oil and Lemon juice	Swallow	½ cup oil plus juice of 1 Lemon	Take in evening
	Camomile	Tea	1 T/cup 4 times/day	works best with 2 Senna pods
		Enema	1 T/cup in enema bag	works best with 2 Senna pods
CONTUSIONS AND BRUISING	Calendula	Tea	1 tsp/cup	
		Compresses		

Comfrey	Tea Compresses	1 tsp/cup	
Willow or Birch	Tea Compress	1 tsp/cup	
Arnica	Homeopathic Tincture	10 drops in ½ cup water	Use every ½ hour until condition is relieved, then less often
DIARRHEA			
Blackberry stem and bark	Infusion		Sip continually until condition is relieved; supplement with Activated Charcoal tablets, 1 / hour, if necessary
Raspberry	Infusion		
Sage	Infusion		
EARS			
Garlic oil, diluted	capsule		Squeeze a Garlic oil perle directly into ear
Mullein flowers	Infusion		
Mullein oil	By dropper	3 drops/ear	

Complaint	Plant	Form of Application	Dose	Additional Information
EARS	Golden Seal and Echinacea	Capsules	2 caps., 3 times/day	Use for 10 days at a time maximum
		Tincture	10 drops 3 times/day	Use for 10 days at a time maximum
EYES	Golden Seal	Wash from a tincture	10 drops/cup of water	
	Comfrey root and Fennel seed	Wash	1 T each herb/cup of water	Can be used as often as necessary
	Camomile	Wash	1 tsp/cups water	Can be used as often as necessary
FUNGUS INFECTIONS	Garlic	Compress Poultice		3 times/day 3 times/day
	Sage	Poultice Tea	1 tsp/cup of water	3 times/day 3 times/day
	Thyme	Poultice Tea		3 times/day 3 times/day

	Golden Seal and Echinacea	Capsules	2 caps., 3 times/day

GALL BLADDER: see LIVER

INFLUENZA: see VIRUS

INSOMNIA	Valerian	Tincture	10 drops once
		Tea	1 tsp/cup
		Homeopathy	2 tablets
	Camomile	Tea	1 tsp/cup of water
		Tincture	10 drops/½ cup water
		Homeopathy	2 tablets
	Orange flowers	Water as a drink	
		Tea	1 tsp/cup

KIDNEYS AND BLADDER	Rose	Tea	Mix all herbs Use 1 T/cup of water
	Alfalfa	Tea	Drink 3 cups/day

Complaint	Plant	Form of Application	Dose	Additional Information
KIDNEYS AND BLADDER	Uva Ursi	Tea		
	Horsetail	Tea		
	Parsley	Tea		
	Marshmallow Root	Tea		
	Sandalwood oil	Inhalation	2 drops at a time	Use Aroma–Vera diffusor
LIVER AND GALLBLADDER	Sage	Tea Culinary	Mix all the herbs Use 1 T/cup of water Drink 3 cups/day	
	Dandelion	Infusion		
	Parsley	Infusion Culinary		
	Kelp	Tea Culinary		
	Rosemary	Tea Culinary		

MENSTRUATION AND WOMEN'S HORMONES	Golden Seal and Echinacea	Capsules	2 capsules 3 times/day
	Rosemary	Infusion Douche Culinary	
	Licorice	Tea Douche	1 tsp/cup drunk hot
	Parsley	Injection	2 fresh sprigs in vagina when period expected
	Rose petals and hips	Tea Bath Compress	
	Rose oil	Inhalation	2 drops at a time
	Sage	Infusion Bath Compress	

Complaint	Plant	Form of Application	Dose	Additional Information
MENSTRUATION AND WOMEN'S HORMONES	Angelica or Dong Quai	Infusion Douche Capsules Bath	6/day	
	Camomile	Infusion Douche		
NERVES AND HEADACHE	Valerian	Tea Compress	1 tsp/cup	Mix the tea herbs Use 1 T mixed herbs/cup of water Drink 3 cups/day
	Spearmint	Infusion Compress		
	Camomile	Tea Compress Bath		
	Lavender	Tea Compress Bath		
	Rosemary	Tea Compress Bath		

Complaint	Plant	Form of Application	Dose	Additional Information
	Alfalfa	Tea Compress		
	Red Clover	Tea Compress		
PAIN (from internal organs): See also the individual organs	Lavender	Infusion		
	White Willow or Birch leaves	Infusion Compress Poultice		
	Marshmallow root	Infusion Compress Poultice		
	Comfrey root	Infusion Compress Poultice		
SICKNESS WITH VOMITING AND STOMACH AILMENTS	Peppermint Oil	Drops Tincture		
	Peppermint	Tea	1 tsp/cup of water	Sip every 15 mins
	Camomile	Tea		

Complaint	Plant	Form of Application	Dose	Additional Information
SORE THROAT	Thyme	Gargle	As needed	Use an infusion
	Comfrey	Gargle	As needed	Use an infusion
	Violet flowers	Gargle Compress	As needed continually	Use an infusion
	Sage	Gargle Compress	As needed	
VIRUS	Rose hips	Infusion	½ cup every 2 hours	steep in covered pot
	Golden Seal and Echinacea	Infusion Capsules	2 every 4 hours	no more than 10 days
	Cayenne	Capsules Tea with Lemon	2 every 4 hours ½ tsp/cup	
	Lemon juice and peel	Decoction Fresh juice		
	Violet flowers	Infusion		

WOUNDS (help healing)	Calendula	Compress Ointment
	Thyme	Compress Tea
	Comfrey root	Compress Ointment Tea
	Marshmallow root	Tea Compress Ointment
	Camomile	Tea Compress Ointment
	Saint John's Wort	Ointment or oil Compress

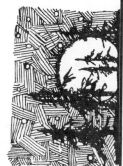

3

...

Mothering

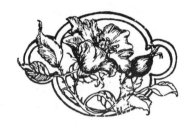

PREPARING FOR BIRTH

Prepare for the birth of your child as though you were training for an athletic event. It's like climbing Mount Everest—you cannot overprepare. Prepare your body, your mind, and your spirit. Learn everything you can about the birth process so that you allay *all* your fears. Fear is the worst enemy in giving birth.

Nowadays there are so many wonderful books and classes to help you get ready for childbirth that there is no excuse for entering parenthood unprepared. There are three things I would like to stress from my own experience as a mother and from the extensive discussions I've had with Nan Koehler, a close friend and a wonderful midwife.

Relaxation. If you can control and relax your body, you will be able to concentrate on the birth process with a sense of pleasure, rather than on your own tension.

Education. Look at pictures and read positive birthing stories to learn the range of experiences that may occur. That way you will be able to visualize where you are in your labor and not fear what is to come.

Preparation. When you can relax the pelvic floor at will, the baby will have no trouble coming out.

Good preparation results in a good birthing experience, which automatically ensures a good bonding experience with your baby. Bonding is Mother Nature's way of making sure you take good care of your child. A mother and child who are well bonded become telepathic. The mother always knows when her baby is hungry and when it needs to be changed, and the baby does not have to become hysterical in order to get proper care.

Bonding is much more intense at home. In a home birth, neither you nor the baby is drugged, and you can have your baby with you immediately. Even if something should go wrong, you are consicously involved in the whole process and you are *still* with your baby. This is one reason I am such a strong advocate of home birth.

A mother properly bonded to her baby will always have a gut-level connection with that child. She will feel it when her child is in a disharmonious situation and will want to do something about it. I have hopes that a whole generation of mothers having natural and home births will be a strong force in changing our society.

HERBS AND PREGNANCY

The use of herbs goes hand in hand with natural birth. Special motivation is needed to go back to the old ways and learn our grandmothers' skills at herbal simples and home remedies. The woman who takes the trouble to learn the use of herbs almost always has a good outcome to her pregnancy.

In preparing herbal teas, it is important not to use any metal. Herbs contain alkaloids that will bind with metal ions in a stainless steel, iron, or aluminum pot or in a metal spoon or tea strainer. The method I use is to measure the herbs into a quart-size glass jar, pour boiling water over them, cover, and let steep. I then sip from the jar all day. If you wish to strain your teas, a bamboo strainer can be used.

There are many herbs that have been used in traditional cultures to aid every stage of the birth process. Those of us reviving the use of herbal simples have found these traditional remedies to be quite effective.

First of all, if you are having trouble *getting* pregnant, there are herbs that will regulate your cycle and tone your endocrine system. Herbs like Sarsaparilla, Licorice root, Gota Kola, Fenugreek, Blessed Thistle, and Squaw Vine are used to strengthen the female reproductive system. Make a quart of tea blended from these herbs and sip throughout the day. In addition, follow an alkaline diet supplemented with vitamins and minerals. You can also take adrenal and pituitary extracts, available at health food stores. Agnus castus is a superior herb for the regulation of pituitary output.

Once you are pregnant, Red Raspberry leaf is the number-one herb to use as a daily tea. Red Raspberry leaf has been used by almost every American Indian tribe as a preparation for childbirth. It is also nutritious and a rich source of minerals. First thing every morning drink a cup of Red Raspberry leaf tea. During the last month of your pregnancy, make a quart of it and sip it throughout the day.

Herbs such as Pennyroyal, Black Cohosh, Blue Cohosh, and Squaw Vine are ecbolics, which means they stimulate Braxton-Hicks contractions. These are the practice muscle contractions of the uterus that ripen your cervix and prepare you for birth. The more Braxton-Hicks contractions you have before labor, the easier your labor will be. A good herbal combination tea to take during the last month of pregnancy would be Red Raspberry leaf, Pennyroyal, Squaw Vine, Skullcap, and Blessed Thistle and Black Cohosh. You don't need to take a lot, just a little throughout the day to keep up the Braxton-Hicks contractions.

You don't have to worry that use of ecbolic herbs will make your baby come prematurely. These herbs will not make your body do anything it's not ready to do by itself. Before you can go into labor, your body must go through a hormonal shift. A surge of prostaglandins, usually a day or two before labor starts, completes the ripening of your cervix, allowing it to open easily. This is why induction of labor doesn't always work. A woman may be having regular contractions, but if she has not had a rise in prostaglandins to soften the cervix, it will not open. Evening Primrose oil may be taken at this time to encourage the surge in prostaglandins.

You may notice that at times during pregnancy your whole body becomes preoccupied with its sensual nature. Having babies is really a very sensual experience. Basil is the herb of choice for you at these times. As you become more familiar with Basil, as a tea and in your cooking, you will feel an attraction to it. It has the kind of energy you want to emulate.

One other way to use herbs during pregnancy is as nutritional supplements. Borage, Comfrey, Nettles, Alfalfa, and Marshmallow root are all rich sources of minerals and can be taken daily with benefit.

VITAMINS

The decision to use vitamins will depend on whether this is your first, second, or third pregnancy. Each time you are pregnant it is a greater strain on your body. If you want to feel really good, be able to function well, and keep your appetite under control, then use vitamins.

Supplements are also necessary because the foods we rely on for vitamins and minerals are grown on depleted soils. Wheat grown on nitrogen-depleted soil is much lower in protein than it should be. Salad greens, normally the best source of folic acid, vitamin A, vitamin C, and minerals, are very poor in nutrients when grown with artificial fertilizers. Ordinarily, milk is an excellent food, but pasteurization destroys its B vitamins and alters the protein. Everywhere we turn the food we rely on for nourishment is no longer nourishing.

If you have no energy, are nervous and irritable, or have irrational food cravings, you need vitamins. Usually, you crave the thing your body needs least! For example, a craving for potato chips, which are very salty, indicates a need for minerals or vitamin A. A craving for sugar means you are deficient in protein or the B vitamins.

Probably the most important supplement to take when you are pregnant is iron, preferably in chelated form. Chelation means the iron is bound to a carbon compound. You can also find iron chelated with amino acids, but the citrated form of iron is the most easily absorbed, because it's the form found naturally in green leafy vegetables. The best source of that type of iron I've found is Dr. Bronner's Calcium Food. It is made of flaked vegetables, such as Carrots and Parsley, and is an excellent and easily absorbed source of iron and calcium. If you are going to take an iron supplement, take at least 70 milligrams daily, along with 2 milligrams of folic acid. If you do this, your tissues will stretch well throughout pregnancy, and you will not tear or bleed much at birth.

You will also need to take vitamin C. In the beginning, take 2 grams (2,000 milligrams) of C daily, increasing to 4–6 grams (4,000–6,000 milligrams) toward the end. Vitamin C helps your body absorb both iron and calcium.

Calcium and magnesium supplements in a ratio of 2:1 will prevent leg cramps, nervous aching, muscle twitching, and insomnia. You should take 2,000 milligrams of calcium and 1,000 of magnesium per day in the evening. Nature's Plus puts out a good calcium/magnesium supplement.

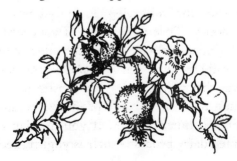

Vitamins E and A are also important. Vitamin E is an antiox-idant and helps your skin stretch. It also helps your body create the hormones that support your pregnancy and keep your body functioning well. Take 1,000 IU per day before bed. Vitamin A will help you avoid colds and is important for proper liver function. Take vitamin A daily in the morning with your B vitamins.

B vitamins are also very important for proper liver function and help prevent nervousness and insomnia. Take a 100-milli-gram-strength B complex tablet daily at breakfast.

In addition to calcium and magnesium, you might want to take a mineral supplement that contains trace minerals such as zinc, manganese, chromium, and all the others that should be in the salad greens you buy at the store but aren't.

All vitamin supplements should be taken in the morning at breakfast, and minerals such as calcium, magnesium, and zinc should be taken at night before bed.

DIET

In general, Nan feels that the healthiest diet to follow when pregnant is a vegetarian or near-vegetarian diet. Read *Diet for a Small Planet,* by Francis Moore Lappe, and *Laurel's Kitchen,* by Laurel Robertson, Carol Flinders, and Bronwen Godfrey, for information on combining grains, seeds, nuts, and legumes to make complete protein meals. If you follow this type of diet, your body will manifest beautifully during your pregnancy.

What I find works best is to focus on the protein and vegeta-ble foods. Avoid the following carbohydrates completely: wheat, sugar, honey. Throw them out of your kitchen—you'll be happier. Minimize salt, take it off the table and learn to taste foods as they really are. Use *The Herbal Guide to Inner Health* for herbal mixtures that will serve as salt substitutes.

Another thing to avoid is dairy products, because they will make you gain too much weight. If you use dairy foods, aim for the fermented dairy products such as yogurt, kefir, and kefir cheese. If you must drink milk, try to get goat's milk as pasteurized cow's milk is a poor food and will make you fat. If you can't give up cow's milk, limit yourself to one cup per day. Cottage cheese, however, should be eliminated from your diet, especially if you have a tendency toward toxemia.

I would like to encourage everyone to learn about the edible wild green things that grow at the edges of gardens and lawns. Malva, Miner's Lettuce, Sow Thistle, Chickweed, Garden Cress, Purslane, and Comfrey are rich sources of folic acid, vitamin C, vitamin A and minerals, much richer than domesticated salad greens. These greens can be chopped up very finely (no one will notice them) and mixed in with your regular salad vegetables. When you do buy salad greens, remember that the deeper the green, the richer the folic acid, vitamins, and minerals. By these standards iceberg lettuce is a waste of money. Why buy it?

When eating fruits, remember not to combine them with vegetables or proteins. Serve fruit in the morning, between meals or a half hour after supper, as a dessert. Since it seems that many women have trouble digesting oranges, it is best to avoid them.

Another good rule is to avoid eating too much of any one thing. Aim for variety. Every day eat seven different kinds of vegetables and a different kind of fruit. This will help you achieve a balanced diet.

Finally, throughout your pregnancy drink plenty of water— at least two quarts per day. If your body is well hydrated when you go into labor, you will have good contractions, and your baby will not get jaundice.

SYMPTOMS AND REMEDIES

One of the earliest symptoms of pregnancy is nausea. Peach leaf, Red Raspberry leaf, Peppermint and Camomile will help bring relief. Since these herbs work best when taken *before* you feel nauseated, you will have to learn to anticipate the symptom. If you tend to feel nauseated in the morning, have a cup of herb tea brought to you in bed and sip before you get up. Or make the tea before bedtime and sip it cold as soon as you awake.

Nausea may be caused by elevated estrogen levels in the body. When you are first pregnant the ovaries secrete extra progesterone and estrogen to support the pregnancy. If you have a weak liver, it can't break down the estrogen fast enough to prevent the suppression of cortisone secretion. And when the cortisone level goes down, your blood sugar level goes down and you feel nauseated. If you have weak adrenals *and* a weak liver, you may experience nausea. Again, take Agnus Castus to encourage more balance in the pituitary hormones.

The best remedy for nausea is B vitamins. The B complex helps your liver function, which prevents chronic elevated estrogen.

Another way to control low blood sugar is to eat 5 or 6 small meals rather than 3 big ones. Carry a snack of fruit, nuts, or seeds and nibble throughout the day to keep blood sugar up. Really focus on eating good-quality, high-protein meals, especially for breakfast. Last thing at night have a high-protein snack. Protein is metabolized very slowly into glucose, which is then slowly released into your bloodstream. For this reason, eating protein keeps your blood sugar level even.

Nausea may also be due to fatigue or stress. If you are nauseated first thing in the morning, it may be that you are not getting enough sleep.

Some women experience insomnia, especially in the third trimester when the baby is getting really big. If this happens to you, make sure you're getting enough calcium, magnesium, B vitamins, and vitamin C. And if you still have trouble, herbal teas can work wonders. Camomile is a mild relaxing herb. Skullcap is a stronger relaxant and Valerian root is stronger still. I find that Ginger Root works best for me, even though Ginger is usually classed as a stimulant. Experiment with these herbs to find the one that works best for you.

BODY CARE

Throughout your pregnancy you will want to oil your stomach to keep from getting stretch marks. Olive oil is the best, but any cold-pressed oil will work well. Pure vitamin E oil can be irritating to the skin, and your cold-pressed oil naturally contains E. You can add an essential oil for scent, or soak fragrant herbs in the vegetable oil. My *Herbal Body Book* is full of recipes for making your own herbals and scented body oils.

One of the best body preparations I have found came from an old black midwife from the South. Her advice was to oil your belly twice a day, morning and evening. Rub the oil around and around clockwise, as hard as you can, then rub it counterclockwise. Then, with a swoop of the hand, oil your labia. This will toughen your vaginal tissues and prepare them for birth. As she put it, "Keep yourself greased up and your baby will just slide right on out."

To prepare your breasts for nursing you can oil your nipples twice a day or roughen them with a towel. Also, going without a bra will desensitize your nipples by letting them rub against your clothes.

One of the most important parts of preparing your body for birth is to prepare your Kegel muscle (the pelvic-floor muscle). A woman who has a naturally loose pelvic floor will have an easy time birthing. But women who are athletic, or who are dancers, have a stronger, thicker perineum and will have to work at being able to relax it.

Actually, every woman should learn to control the Kegel muscle. The instinctive reaction when you feel the baby's head pushing on the pelvic floor is to tighten the Kegel muscle. The pressure of the baby's head stimulates the rectal nerves, creating the sensation of having a bowel movement. And we have all been so effectively toilet trained that before we know it we have tensed the Kegel muscle. With good Kegel control you can consciously let loose, the muscle will relax, and your uterus can then easily push the baby out.

To practice controlling your Kegel muscle: tighten it, tighten it, tighten it, and then release. Do this many times every day. You can reach such a degree of control that you can ripple the muscle from front to back and back to front, and close your anal sphincter without closing your urethra!

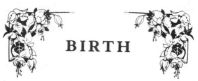

BIRTH

LABOR

If you wake up in the morning with regular contractions, chances are good you will have your baby later that day. If your labor starts in the evening, ignore it. More than likely it's false labor. As you get closer to your due date, fatigue at the end of the day will set off Braxton-Hicks contractions. Many women will get regular contractions after supper and stay up all night, thinking they are in labor. The best thing to do is drink a relaxing herbal tea and go to sleep. If you really *are* in labor, the pains will wake you up toward morning, and you will at least have had some rest.

When you do finally go into labor, make sure you eat a good, solid, high-protein meal—something to sustain you. Also, since the same nerves innervate both the lower intestines and the uterus, you stimulate your contractions by eating. After you have eaten, go for a good 2- or 3-mile hike. When you come home, take a nice hot bath and relax. Your labor should be coming along just fine by now.

A good birthing tea to drink at this point is made of equal parts Basil, Lavender, Nutmeg, and Red Raspberry leaf. Make a mild tea (it's bitter if too strong) and drink a pot or two, sipping between contractions. An obstetrician friend of mine has been very impressed with how effective this tea is for stimulating labor. I have found that standard birthing herbs such as Pennyroyal, Black Cohosh, and Blue Cohosh stimulate contractions but will not actually bring on your labor.

If your membranes rupture early and you are only in mild labor, it is important to birth the baby as soon as possible. The best herbal home remedy for this purpose is good old Castor oil. Drink four ounces of it straight down on an empty stomach. Soon afterward you will have violent diarrhea, your contractions will start, and your baby will be born a few hours later. Because it is a strong purgative, Castor oil stimulates your lower intestines and uterus just as eating does, only much more powerfully. It takes a strong-willed knowledgeable woman to drink Castor oil when it is so easy to take Pitocin, but for a *natural* birth, Castor oil is the method of choice. It is safe. If your membranes were to rupture 3 weeks before the baby was due, Castor oil would not force a labor that wasn't already underway.

If your labor is moving very slowly, you may have low blood sugar or be dehydrated. Eat something and drink several glasses of diluted fruit juice or herbal tea. The birthing tea mentioned above may help here too.

Sometimes labor is slowed by tension—either muscular or nervous. Oil of Celery, available at health food stores, is a powerful muscle relaxant. The dose is 7–10 drops in a glass of water, taken between contractions. Sometimes a woman needs to cry in order to release tension, especially if she has any fear of becoming a mother.

Another wonderful way to help labor along is to get into a tub of hot (herbal) water. This is especially useful if your legs and bottom are tense, which in turn tightens up the Kegel muscle. Sometimes a woman in labor needs to be alone, to concentrate on what is happening in her own body without worrying about anyone else. A bathtub is a good place to be alone, to relax and focus on letting the baby come out. Also, water is cleansing to the spirit. In all religions, water is used to purify. During birth, a water bath can help you ground yourself and purify your energy.

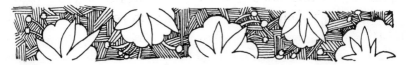

BIRTH AND AFTERBIRTH

Once the baby is actually coming out, the best way to prevent tearing is to birth the head quite slowly so the perineum has time to stretch. The perineal tissue is very elastic, but will tear if you stretch it too fast. As the baby's head becomes visible, oil the head and the labia with Olive oil. It's best not to actually touch the perineum—just drip the oil on it at the point of maximum stretch, which will keep the tissue moist and elastic. Often it will tear *just* where you touch it.

As soon as the baby comes out of the woman's body, put it on her belly or between her breasts. It is somehow important to the bonding process to have the baby there, hot and wet, where the woman can smell, touch, and see this "fruit" of her body. If you need to work on the baby, you can do it just as well on her abdomen as on the bed. As soon as the placenta emerges and the cord is cut, have your birthing attendant position the baby for nursing. It is important to nurse the baby as soon as possible as the sucking reflex is strongest right after birth.

You do not need to leave the responsibility for the afterbirth to your birthing attendant. Make a mental note after you push the baby out that you will have two more contractions, three to five minutes apart. The first one detaches the placenta from the uterus, with the second you push the placenta out. If the placenta does not come within ten to fifteen minutes, squat over a bowl and push it out. It will come out easily. Then lie back in bed and massage the top of your uterus to keep it hard and prevent excessive bleeding. The herb to use now is Angelica root. This herb, which you can buy in tincture form, has been used by the Indians from ancient times to help with the expulsion of the placenta. To prevent excessive bleeding, I like to use Cayenne pepper powder in capsules. Shepherd's purse is also good for bleeding, but does not work when dried. If you do not have the fresh plant growing abundantly in your garden try to start some.

CARE OF THE NEWBORN

NURSING

The best way to keep your breasts functioning well without any trouble from cracked nipples is to nurse the baby continually from the moment of birth. And I mean continually. Every time the baby rouses, nurse it and keep on nursing. By the time your milk comes in on the second or third day, all your colostrum will be milked out and your breasts won't get engorged. When your breasts are engorged, the baby can't grip the nipple properly and it cracks. Engorgement is caused by a prolactin surge on the third day after birth when the gonadotrophin hormone is finally metabolized out of your body. There is a sudden and intense flow of blood to the milk-making tissues of the breast, which lasts for 24 to 48 hours. If you keep the breasts well drained at this time the engorgement subsides and you will have no trouble with your nipples.

In general, you should follow the same good nutrition program while nursing that you did when you were pregnant. Remember that your baby can only be as healthy as your milk. If there are problems, treat them through your milk. If the baby is dehydrated, *you* drink more water. If the baby gets sick often, *you* need more vitamins. If you want to give the baby herbs, *you* drink the herb tea. Exceptions are colic, gas, and indigestion, for which a little pure acidophilus culture can be given directly to improve the baby's intestinal flora.

MOTHERING

Often a really colicky baby is the result of something the mother is doing—a bitter pill for some women to swallow. My baby is me. If my baby is fussy, it means I'm fussy. Perhaps I'm upset about something and my milk won't let down or my touch doesn't soothe. Or perhaps my timing in taking care of the baby is off. Often, 4:00 to 6:00 P.M. is the baby's most social time, and it will then have trouble quieting down for sleep.

Often the baby will cry and cry until it falls asleep from sheer exhaustion. If you learn to catch this cycle before the baby gets too excited—give it a bath or take it out into the fresh air—you will have a calm baby.

One of the arts of mothering is burping your baby thoroughly. Otherwise, care of a baby is really simple. If the baby fusses or cries, take care of it. Change it whenever it is wet and nurse it all the time. If it doesn't like one breast, give it the other. Make sure your baby gets enough sleep. Bathe the baby daily and make sure that all cloth next to the baby's skin is 100 percent cotton and clean, soft, and dry. Carry your baby around with you at all times. There have been many studies showing that motion keeps babies happy and healthy—it helps them digest their food and breathe properly. You can strap the baby to your body, which lets you do your work and keep the baby in motion as you move about.

I would like to end with something you will not read in any other book. If your baby has difficulty centering in its body, if it is lethargic, sleeps too much, or rolls its eyes around—give a series of hot Rosemary baths. Make the bath by boiling Rosemary herb in water and straining the brew into the bathtub. When it reaches the proper temperature, float the baby in the hot Rosemary water. Do this two or three times and your baby will be a transformed being.

It's magical the way herbs can work.

For those who would like more information, I suggest reading *Artemis Speaks: VBAC Stories and Natural Childbirth Information,* by Nan Ullrike Koehler (available from Jerald R. Brown, Inc., 17440 Taylor Lane, Occidental, CA 95465.

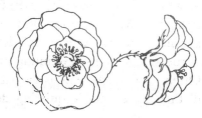

4
· · ·
The Herbal
Child

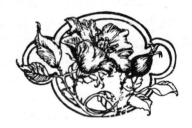

Children can be raised naturally and herbally. Perhaps because of inexperience there is a tendency for mothers to depend too much on the advice of others (usually an M.D.). If we listen to our feelings, our intuitions, and the words of *one* older and more experienced person, we can raise a child without resorting to harsh chemicals, drugs, or frightening surgery. When children become sick, they need love and tenderness above anything else.

For instance, a child with an earache can sleep if the mother will do only two simple things. First, squeeze a perle of Garlic oil (Garlic infused in vegetable oil) into each ear and then bundle the child up warmly and sit in a rocking chair with the aching ear pressed against your body, rocking quietly and rhythmically until the child sleeps. (See Chapter 2 for more information on Garlic.)

This is only one example of how love and attention and a little herbal knowledge can help to quickly terminate a potentially dangerous situation in which the child could become really sick. But if you just give the child a tablet of aspirin and tell him or her to sleep and that you will go to see the doctor in the morning, you only increase the likelihood of the child's becoming sick. The Garlic oil and the rocking chair will do more healing and helping than the aspirin ever could.

DIET

The child should be encouraged to eat fruits and vegetables and to go lightly on meats and whole grains during a stressful time of potential sickness. Children have a tendency to eat bread and butter or bread and Peanut butter to the exclusion of anything else. Offer a fresh crisp salad first at every meal and then the Potatoes and grains. Children often like special things in their salad; it could be Avocadoes or it could be shrimp. But whatever it is, as long as it is wholesome, be sure to offer it. My son loves whole Wheat bread and hummus or Peanut butter. This is a wholesome combination of foods, but he will often eat these grains and neglect his greens. Our alternative is to feed him another favorite, Pasta al Pesto. The sauce is crammed full of fresh raw greens and can be used over pasta, bread, or baked Potatoes. He especially likes the narrow green noodles made with whole Wheat and Spinach with this green sauce.

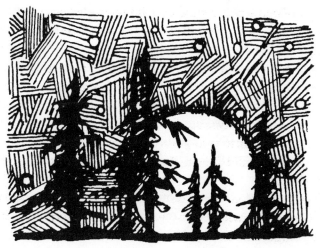

PESTO SAUCE

Approximate ingredients

1/4	cup Olive oil
1	cup fresh chopped Basil or Parsley or combination
1/4–1/2	cup Pinon nuts or Almonds
1/4–1/2	cup or more Parmesan cheese
3	cloves Garlic
	dash fresh Pepper
	some salt
	dash Cayenne

Chop the greens and the Garlic. Put into a blender and add a bit of Olive oil. Blend on low speed. From time to time stop the blender to push down the ingredients with a rubber spatula. Add the Pinon nuts and blend. Mix in the Parmesan cheese and the spices. The end consistency should be like thick crunchy Peanut butter.

EAR CARE

Some children, including my son Bryan, have a weakness in their ears that seems to encourage ear infections and earaches. These children with their short ear canals should never be given swimming lessons before the age of 5 or 6. Most children have short ear canals but do not necessarily have ear infections. Look to yourself: As a child did you have many earaches? If so, think before signing up your child for swimming lessons. I had earaches as a child, but thinking that Bryan should learn to swim at an early age, I enrolled him in swimming lessons when he was 8 months old. And this was in August, which is often cold and foggy here in San Francisco. Without any protection, such as filling his ears with a good lubricating oil like Garlic or Mullein, I put him in the heavily chlorinated water daily for 5 days. By the week's end he had an earache that came and went regularly for the next 2 years.

During this time I developed the following treatment that worked on him as well as on other children who tried it. Since that time he has never had an earache.

Mulleined Oil is made by steeping Mullein flowers in Olive oil. Fill a small jar with the flowers and add a good-quality Olive oil. Cover and let steep for 2 weeks. Strain the oil through clean cheesecloth and store it in a lightproof sterile bottle.

Mullein flower tincture is made by filling a small jar with Mullein flowers and covering the flowers with a high-quality clear alcohol, such as 100 proof vodka. Let this mixture steep for 2 weeks, then strain through clean cheesecloth into a small bottle and store the tincture until it is needed.

Before swimming or exposure put 3–4 drops of the Mulleined oil into each ear and massage around the outside of the ear to make sure the oil penetrates all the way down into the canal.

After swimming or exposure, dilute 10 drops of the tincture with 10–20 drops of water and put half of the diluted tincture into each ear, being careful to massage it in.

About once a week wash out the ears carefully using an ear syringe and a catch basin. Use a warm, carefully strained infusion of Mullein flowers, Comfrey root, and Marshmallow root: about ½ ounce of the mixed herbs to 2 cups of water. Suck the liquid up into the ear syringe and squeeze into the ear, catching the overflow in the catch basin. Continue until the liquid is used up; alternate in each ear. If you intend to wash a child's ears, always try out the solution on yourself first. You need to know exactly how warm the liquid is and with what strength you will need to squeeze the bulb. Never do anything to a child that you have not first tried on yourself. This Mullein earwash is also excellent for children with hard, sticky earwax or children who may have collected sand in their ears. Wax and sand create a deadly mixture that forms a sort of scratchy concrete in the ear and becomes a source of bacterial infection. Adults as well as children will benefit from this earwash.

The washing is healing and it cleans hard wax and debris from the ear canal; the oil protects before exposure, while the alcohol acts as an antiseptic and evaporates any water that may have entered the canals while swimming. This ear care method can be used on any earache, not just swimmer's ear.

CARING FOR A SICK CHILD

How do you as a parent know when your child is sick? Do you regularly look at his or her eyes, checking for circles or that certain tightness in the skin that occurs *before* a child is sick? Do you look at the skin and check for sallowness, paleness, or a redness to the cheeks? Do you check the way the child is walking or talking or acting? Often a child will be cranky and irritable several days before he or she actually comes down with anything. Do you smell the child's body? A sick person, though he or she may have no outward symptoms, will often smell sickly sweet or sour before being reduced to lying in bed. All the secretions of the body, from nose mucus to sweat to urine and feces, may develop a strange "off" odor before the child is obviously sick. If you will look at all these signs and keep the child home for a day or two before he or she is actually, unmistakably sick you will often be able to prevent serious illness. Provide a diet heavy on vegetable juices and fruits and light on protein and grain carbohydrates. Give plenty of vitamin C, especially the controlled time release type, as well as good doses of B vitamins, vitamins A and E, and the minerals zinc and calcium. Let the child rest in bed playing quietly, keep the child surrounded with soft, muted colors, and for heaven's sake do not give sugary pop, ice cream or other such sick "treats."

If you have followed all these directions and your child still gets sick, look for the following signs. Take the child's temperature, because fever is often a side effect of childhood illnesses. Fever is a way for the body to burn up a virus. Therefore, do not necessarily try to bring it down. It must only be brought down if there is a danger of convulsion. My favorite way to reduce fever is to run a body-temperature bath with an infusion of Melilot in the water. Into the bath goes the feverish child with some favorite bath toy. Often I add epsom salts to the bath to help bring toxins to the surface of the skin. Cold water is slowly run into the bath to reduce the water's temperature. I play with the child in the tub and watch carefully so that he or she does not begin to chill.

When the child or baby has been in the tub for 10–15 minutes, remove and wrap in a 100 percent cotton terrycloth towel. It is my belief that polyester in any fabric is an energy drain for humans. Consequently I do not use it, not under any circumstances. Wrap the child loosely in the towel and let him or her put on some loose cotton pajamas. Then you can put the child to bed, remembering not to cover too heavily but making sure that the room is draft-free and comfortable. A feverish child should be given as much liquid—water or weak tea—as he or she will drink so that there will be no danger of dehydration. My son would never drink when he was sick, so I would sit him in my lap for hours at a time, giving him weak solutions of Camomile tea, Mullein flower tea, or an appropriate tea by drops from an eye dropper.

A hot-air vaporizer is inexpensive and a very helpful addition to the sickroom. Put it somewhere where the vapors will reach the child but where it will be safe from overturning. Add an essential oil, such as Sandalwood or Cinnamon, to the well of the vaporizer, choosing the oil appropriate for the illness. Let the vaporizer run all the time the child sleeps. This keeps an essential oil constantly medicating a sick person. I use an Aroma-Vera diffusor, available from Aroma-Vera in Culver City, CA.

I use Eucalyptus oil as an antiseptic and for colds and runny noses, Sandalwood oil when the kidneys need to be worked on, Peppermint oil when there is a "hot" fever, and Cinnamon oil when the fever is the cold and clammy type. Mixtures of oils are also suitable—for example, a mixture of Basil and Eucalyptus for blocked sinus, or Lavender and Spearmint as an antispasmodic for asthma.

Check the pulse rate of the child often to determine the severity of the illness. Irregular pulse is often a very serious sign and a doctor should be sought if this is the case. Take the pulse using a watch with a second hand for a full minute and write down the results. *Do not trust your memory.* In fact, it is wise to keep a running record of all the signs and symptoms of your child's illness to help you distinguish the signs of a slight indisposition from those of more serious problems in the future. A pulse of less than 60 is irregular, as is one that is greater than 160.

Check how your child is breathing. Respiratory infections will surely alter the breathing pattern. This is when the vaporizer comes in very handy. In my household we use a vaporizer or diffusor during the winter with antiseptic oils in the well. It smells good and helps to keep airborne germs at a minimum.

Digestive disturbances and many childhood diseases can cause diarrhea and vomiting. In each case keep food simple and light and make sure the child has plenty of liquids. For diarrhea, give only really ripe bananas to eat. Certain homeopathic remedies are excellent as is a drop of Peppermint oil given in a tablespoon of water. The Peppermint oil can be given every few hours. Garlic soup made with chicken broth is an excellent restorative for digestive disturbances of all sorts.

When your child is sick the most important item in his or her recovery is plenty of love and attention from Mom *and* a positive attitude.

A few weeks ago on the night before my son and I were to leave on a long-anticipated trip to Colorado to see the Rockies, he suddenly became feverish, with sore achy ears. I told him that he had to think himself well and happy because if he woke up sick he would have to stay home. I read to him that evening some particularly positive, pleasant children's stories, gave him plenty of vitamin C, dropped Garlic oil from perles into his ears, and let him sleep with me in my bed, all the while repeating how well he felt and especially how terrific he would feel when he woke up. All this extra attention turned this little boy with the pallor in his skin and the bright red dots on his cheeks into a healthy and happy person in the morning. We took our trip and he never came down with whatever was trying to get him.

This chapter is not meant to teach you how to treat all childhood diseases or any in particular, only to help you with the general signs and symptoms of illness.

My favorite treatments and herbs for children are herb baths, the use of the diffusor with essential oils, always dressing the child in natural fabrics, and providing simple, nutritious foods with an abundance of vegetables and fruits.

INTERNAL CARE

For all their seeming toughness, children are new to this earth and can have delicate constitutions. Their skin is sensitive and you should be extra careful that the products you use with them are delicate and made with care. My favorite all-purpose remedy is a mixture of Calendula (Marigold), Camomile, and Comfrey. These 3 herbs start with the letter C, as does the word children, and this is a simple way to remember the herbs. If you will make an infusion of this mixture (mix equal parts and store) you can use it in half a dozen or more ways: on a child's skin or for a sensitive person as a bath herb mixture; as a tea for any type of respiratory or digestive distress; as external wash for skin conditions or bruises or as a cosmetic wash for the skin or a rinse for the hair. The mixture is excellent to soften your favorite shampoo; it will also lighten and brighten the hair. It can be used as a base for a cream, lotion, or massage oil. Marigold is considered an herb of the sun and the herb of goodness. There is absolutely nothing toxic about the 3-C herbs for children, and they can be used in combination with complete assurance.

Another excellent tonic mixture for children is Rose Petal Elixir. This can be made at home or it can be purchased from Weleda Products in Spring Valley, New York, or through Herbal Home Products in Rescue, California, both by mail.

EXTERNAL CARE

Children's skin should be taken care of with good soap and water, a soothing cream, a gentle shampoo, and always herbs in the bath. The 3-C children's herb mixture can be used in the bath or as the base for a soothing cream.

LOOK YOUR CHILD OVER EVERY DAY

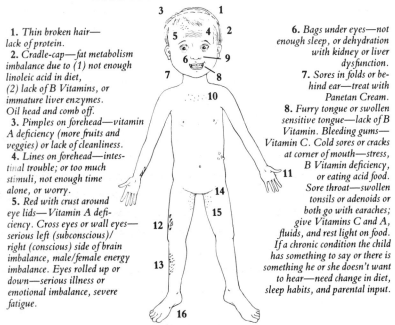

1. *Thin broken hair—lack of protein.*

2. *Cradle-cap—fat metabolism imbalance due to (1) not enough linoleic acid in diet, (2) lack of B Vitamins, or immature liver enzymes. Oil head and comb off.*

3. *Pimples on forehead—vitamin A deficiency (more fruits and veggies) or lack of cleanliness.*

4. *Lines on forehead—intestinal trouble; or too much stimuli, not enough time alone, or worry.*

5. *Red with crust around eye lids—Vitamin A deficiency. Cross eyes or wall eyes—serious left (subconscious)/right (conscious) side of brain imbalance, male/female energy imbalance. Eyes rolled up or down—serious illness or emotional imbalance, severe fatigue.*

6. *Bags under eyes—not enough sleep, or dehydration with kidney or liver dysfunction.*

7. *Sores in folds or behind ear—treat with Panetan Cream.*

8. *Furry tongue or swollen sensitive tongue—lack of B Vitamin. Bleeding gums—Vitamin C. Cold sores or cracks at corner of mouth—stress, B Vitamin deficiency, or eating acid food. Sore throat—swollen tonsils or adenoids or both go with earaches; give Vitamins C and A, fluids, and rest light on food. If a chronic condition the child has something to say or there is something he or she doesn't want to hear—need change in diet, sleep habits, and parental input.*

9. *Blue or swollen inner nose—allergic mucosa (low-grade food allergy).*

10. *Rash on chest—chemical or food allergy, heat rash, or too much citrus fruit, with a fever consider it a cleansing ailment and lighten up on food.*

11. *Fingers and toes correspond to the 5 lower chakras or energy centers of the body. If they are out of place that energy center is out of balance or if one has illnesses in the body at those centers it represents an imbalance: 1 = Earth or grounding on the material plane; 2 = water or feelings; 3 = fire or power; 4 = heart or love; 5 = senses (speech, hearing, etc.); 6 = integration of knowledge or instincts; and 7 = Crown or God consciousness or spirituality or connection with the universe.*

12. *Scabies that crust—impetigo. Wash more often with soap and water. Poultice or plantain and more vitamins.*

13. *Poison Oak—all treatments aim at itc prevention. It will heal in 3 days if no scratching.*

14. *Rashes—urine burns or smegma accumulation or yeast infection. Wash more often and if yeast dab with diluted Apple cider vinegar. Be sure diapers are double-rinsed.*

15. *Pinworms—have child eat 4–6 Nasturtium leaves and again 17 days later.*

16. *Puncture wound—make sure it bleeds, then soak in Apple cider vinegar bath.*

3-C CREAM FOR CHILDREN

1   T Camomile
1   T Comfrey root
1   T Calendula flowers (Marigold)
4   oz Olive oil
     Dab of beeswax (about 1 T)

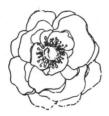

Make a thick infusion of the herbs. Strain out the herbs and add the herbal liquid to the oil. Simmer until most of the water has boiled off. Add the beeswax and heat until it is melted. Remove from the heat and stir until the cream is solid and cooled.

This cream is especially good for burns or irritated mucous passages, or as a diaper rash ointment. My favorite children's soap is Neca 7. This alkali-free baby soap leaves the skin fresh and soft. It is available in many stores or by mail order through Truc, Inc., in Woodstock Hill, Connecticut.

Here is an excellent simple first-aid eyewash recipe that is one of my staples: Simmer 1 tablespoon each of Comfrey root and Fennel seed in 4 ounces of water for a few minutes. Cover the pot, turn off the heat, and steep until cool. Strain carefully through a fine textured fabric, such as an old pair of nylons, and refrigerate. Always keep this formula in the fridge and remake it every 3 days.

INOCULATIONS

Twenty-two years ago, my daughter received all the inoculations then available. When Bryan was born 13 years ago, he got everything except smallpox shots. If I were to have a child now I would carefully read all of the current literature, both from the medical profession and from the alternative health care viewpoint, before I allowed my child to have any inoculations.

Many are of the opinion that the questionable effects of immunizations outweigh the benefits. Children who are raised on a wholesome diet in a sanitary environment probably do not need most of the vaccinations they are given today. Sometimes the vaccine itself can trigger the disease. Often the decline in a disease comes just about the same time as the vaccine and there is often doubt that the vaccine caused the decline. Sometimes the study of the disease leads to the knowledge of how it is contracted and spread and this knowledge leads to the reduction of the disease just about the same time the vaccine is "discovered." In *Confessions of a Medical Heretic* by Robert S. Mendelsohn, M.D., there is more information about the questionable effects of immunizations. This book, published by Warner Books in 1979, is still very much available at bookstores and is fascinating reading.

This is a subject loaded with emotional impact and each parent should investigate all the alternatives before automatically getting inoculations.

CIRCUMCISION

When my son was born his father and I decided that we would not have him circumcised. The pediatrician carefully told us to clean the penis each time he urinated by pulling the skin all the way back from the glans. Any mother who has had a son knows that this is impossible without serious damage to the penis and will cause great harm and pain to the baby whose foreskin is forcibly pushed back from the glans. *So don't pull the skin back.* The skin adheres to the glans just as the peel of an orange adheres to the flesh of the orange. As the boy grows these adhesions will gradually diminish until the skin can be pushed back all the way to reveal the entire glans. Your son will also help in this process, because as he grows he will begin to take an interest in his organs and start to play with them and soon will be pushing on the skin all by himself. Do not discourage him in this type of play. At the same time he will be becoming potty trained and can also be taught to wash his penis at least once a day.

Sometimes material will gather under the skin and cause irritation. This material is called smegma: Wash it away with a gentle soap and plenty of water and then apply a soothing cream such as Bruise Juice from New Age Creations (in San Francisco) or Marigold Flower Balm (from Herbal Home Products, Rescue, CA). Sometimes if the boy forgets to wash or forgets to shake the urine from his penis, the urine will cause an irritation and even redness and swelling. It is important that the boy know what this irritation is, and he should be taught to keep his penis as well as the rest of his body clean and reasonably odor-free.

PUBERTY

When I was 12, I weighed 90 pounds, was shaped rather like a twig, swam every day in the summer, and didn't think much about anything else. Just 6 months later, I weighed 116, was 5 feet 3 inches tall, had hair on my body that needed removing, and had begun to think about formals and dates. Whenever I moved during this horrible period, I bumped into walls and door jambs and stumbled on carpet threads. My appetite and the appetites of my friends, both male and female, were truly awesome. We ate, and ate—three meals a day plus hamburgers and cherry Cokes after school and then pizzas and grilled-cheese sandwiches after dinner. As a girl I was unfamiliar with the problems that a boy might experience, but as a mother I can see the changes that my handsome 14-year-old Bryan is just now beginning to undergo.

My son is experiencing many of the same problems I suffered through at his age. Physically, the body changes—enlarges, lengthens, thickens here, thins there. A girl has menarche, a boy begins to masturbate; they both sprout hair in strange new places. Kids may begin to rebel in school; no longer are they the obedient, "good" kids we once knew. Schoolwork may suffer. Physical changes may temporarily transform a handsome child

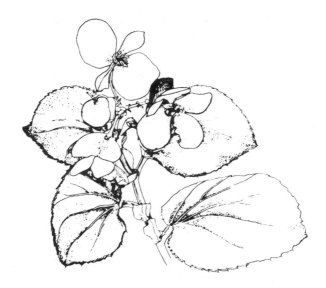

into an awkward tangle of gangly limbs. Sex becomes interesting and dates may become a social requirement. Problems may arise that are of grave importance to parents, such as drugs and drink. But these problems may be of only minor interest to the child, who may be more terrified of "terminal" acne or erupting zits. Eating disorders may arise; and how about lying, stealing, or going steady?

Many of these issues are quite beyond the scope of this book, but several issues can be discussed that will surely simplify the poor parents' life during these trying years.

Generally, boys and girls need information and advice on skin care and body care.

Food supplements should be taken to balance a system that is literally changing daily. Both my children, Amber now 23 and Bryan, 14, have had very little trouble with their skin and their health because I supplemented their diets regularly with nutritional additions. Vitamins and minerals should be taken regularly during puberty. These should include stress items such as folic acid (available in Spinach), zinc, plenty of vitamin C with bioflavonoids (eat Oranges with the white membrane, which contains the bioflavonoids needed to use vitamin C and to strengthen the capillaries and minimize the bruising that occurs in contact sports). Bonemeal is important for calcium levels and bone growth and should be taken at night just before bed. Brewer's yeast can be taken to provide B vitamins and a complete and balanced B complex. One ounce of bee pollen should be taken daily as well.

Herbs during puberty should include the high-calcium herbs such as Borage and Comfrey for growing bones and for menstrual cramps that may occur in young girls experiencing their first menstruation. Girls should also include the woman's root, Angelica, also called Dong Quai, which will balance the hormones and tonify the developing menstrual cycle. Parsley should be given daily to both boys and girls because it contains large amounts of needed nutrients. It also has a cleansing effect on the excretory system, which many kids may need because of the nutritionally deficient foods they eat.

A basic herbal recipe for boys could be Borage, Sarsaparilla, Echinacea and, Parsley; and for a girl, Comfrey, Dong Quai, Echinacea, and Parsley. Equal parts of these herbs can be mixed, using 3 ounces of each herb. Mix them and store in a lightproof container. About ½ ounce of this mixture should be steeped overnight in one quart of water, poured in at just under boiling temperature. In the morning strain this mixture and drink it freely throughout the day. This tea can be drunk throughout puberty. It is a mistake to give the stronger woman's herbs, such as Cohosh or Pennyroyal to a young girl. For a boy, avoid large amounts of Ginseng. The child's system is just developing and doesn't need the violent kick these herbs can give. For both boys and girls, Rosemary, Comfrey, Borage, Parsley, Nettles, Blackberry, Spinach, and Angelica are gentle and much better herbs to use.

Body odor can be a horribly smelly problem. Often it seems that no amount of bathing can solve the body odor of a boy or girl during puberty. This odor is detectable on the breath as well as on the body and has a rather sour, offensive, and pungent vibration. In our household we solved this problem easily. *We simply added clay to the diet.* The edible clays available on the market are tasteless. They absorb toxins and are excreted with the feces. One teaspoon of *green* clay taken in a half glass of water night and morning for 1 week solved our problem completely. The children no longer had any nasty body odor and therefore did not need to use strong antiperspirants nor antibacterial soaps. As we now know after years of experience, these can cause more trouble in the long run than they solve in the present.

The children and young people I am acquainted with who have used the green clay have all had remarkable success, and they've never had to take the treatment for longer than 2 weeks. Also, this treatment rarely had to be repeated. If the body odor begins to return take clay for a few days and lighten the diet to just fruits and vegetables. Along with the clay treatment take tablets of zinc daily as well as more brewer's yeast.

Pimples, blackheads, and oily or dry regions on the adolescent's skin can be handled in various ways but most easily through the use of clay packs. These troubled areas on the skin usually occur where oily hair touches the skin—for example, on the back or face. Naturally, you must exclude sugar and junk food from the diet and increase the amount of raw foods, fruits, and vegetables that is eaten. No amount of vitamin or clay therapy can offset a poor diet. A consistent cleansing program must be initiated that includes washing twice a day using a neutral or bland soap such as Neca 7 or Neutrogena. Skin steaming using a mixture of detoxifying herbs such as Fennel seed, Lavender blossom, and Comfrey root is also effective. This mixture can also be applied as a compress. Clay packs made with red clay (used for blood purification) can be applied daily. The liquid that is mixed with the clay should be Burdock root water, the liquid from your steam mixture, or even a mixture of Apple cider vinegar, Lemon juice, and water, if the skin is especially oily. Directly after the clay packs the skin may be more than usually sensitive and the pimples may be more noticeable until they "head," pop, and drain. They will then scab and eventually disappear. Clay works wonderfully well and the children should not become discouraged when they see that the pimples seem even larger after the clay pack applications. This is the time to pay especial attention to the diet. Eat plenty of nourishing, "clean," wholesome foods and you will even be able to eat "junk" and burgers and still have beautiful skin.

SPECIAL PROBLEMS FOR GIRLS

When my daughter and her friend simultaneously experienced their menarche, I found to my utter amazement that the problems of puberty were nowhere discussed in the hundreds of herbal volumes I have in my library. Menarche is the first menstrual period in a woman's life; puberty is the time in a child's life when the sex organs begin to mature and usually occurs between the ages of 11 and 14. It specifically occurs in a girl when she reaches a weight of 92–102 pounds. This explains why young girls who maintain intensive exercise regimes in which their weight is contained within tight limits often do not go through menarche until they are 15 or 16. Puberty lasts a longer or shorter time depending on the individual.

Puberty in a young girl shows in her narrowing waistline, rounding hips, a new awareness in the eyes and facial expression, a difference in gait, a growth of curly hair on the armpits, legs, and pubic region, a usually rapid growth of the breast tissue, and ultimately, the menarche. The hormones begin to course through the body causing these changes and often creating emotional difficulties in the young girl. Exercise should be vigorous—any games and sports are useful.

Breasts need care and a concerned mother should teach a girl how to massage her growing breasts and hips to minimize the possibility of stretch marks. These remarks could also be noted by pregnant women. Cocoa butter or lanolin can be warmed and used in massage as well as Wheat germ oil scented with oil of Sage. Stretch marks are very difficult or impossible to get rid of once you've got them. So the trick is to *not* get stretch marks in the first place. As the breasts grow, blue lines radiate from the center of the breasts, which can be very tender to the touch. The nipple area enlarges and often itches unmercifully. Put your thumbs on your nipples and cup your palms around the breasts and massage *gently* in a circular motion, using any of the creams or lotions described. The breasts should be massaged once or twice a day until most of the growth is reached.

Vaginal discharge in the young girl (who has not had intercourse) should be handled simply and gently by the use of hip baths containing Comfrey and Rose petals, followed by the application of a gentle cream containing Marigold flowers. A salve or cream can be easily made at home using your own recipe or the one listed on page 67 of *Kitchen Cosmetics,* or you could purchase a Marigold flower salve, such as that made by Herbal Home Products, located in Rescue, California. Weleda, at 30 South Main Street in Spring Valley, NY 10977, sells exquisite Camomile and Marigold cosmetics and that wonderful red clay called Luvos.

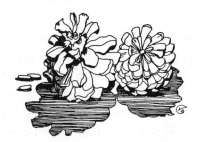

SPECIAL PROBLEMS WITH BOYS

My friend Nan Koehler has several boys. They are all handsome, healthy, seemingly well-adjusted, and self-possessed. Any mother would be proud of boys like these. She recently sent me this letter, which is reproduced in its entirety.

A confounding landmark of childhood is early or preadolescence, the ages 11, 12, 13. By age 10 (the proverbial "plateau of childhood") our child seems to be blossoming; doing well in school, on athletic teams, independent, etc. Suddenly at about age 11 they become demanding, jealous, full of desires, alternately sweet or horrible (hormones are decreasing and then suddenly peaking). Unless we are unusually wise, patient, and experienced (which most of us aren't) the tempest of those years lays the foundation for potential alienation at the mid-teen years. By age 15 your boy will either be pretty sensible or on the road to potentially destructive social/cultural alienation.

Now, how do we catch our child's attention, away from TV, away from flashy clothes, loud music, and the continual stream of friends? How do we catch children's attention when they have been under the influence of school or day care people all day. How can we catch their attention when we see them following a dead-end path or adopting destructive habits such as tobacco smoking, TV addiction, excessive coffee drinking, or alcohol consumption and mindless consumerism?

The technique used for countless generations is called the *rite of passage*. Traditionally held at age 13, this ritual, ceremony, or observance usually included the use of the sacramental herbs. Herbs helped open the mind, provided endurance during physical hardships, and provided the matrix for rebonding with parents during this time when the tribal secrets were passed along. Under the influence of various psychedelics, ritual information was repeatedly sung, drummed, or spoken into the child's ear. This ceremony was not a short one-time, one-hour affair, but a drawn-out process lasting anywhere from three intense days to over a year. The boys were systematically initiated into adult consciousness. They were told what was to be expected of them in *every* situation. This was done in "dream-time," with love, not with a harangue.

We too can do this today with our boys by using sacramental herbs *together* with them, taking them on pilgrimages, taking them to power spots, outdoors, and into the garden. We can include them in adult rituals of all sorts. We can be always available to answer any questions and provide guidance. This is a critical time. This is the time to talk with the 11- to 12-year-old child if we want to teach him the consequences of actions. This talk must be done before age 14; after puberty, the laws of cause and effect can only be learned through experience.

Please don't be afraid to use our sacred earth-bonding herbs *with* your boy.

Use them wisely, use them well, use them together with your son, only during those formative years called puberty. Always be available for conversation, discussion. You never know when your son (or your daughter) is ready to have a serious discussion. Sometimes these "talks" are preceded by all sorts of hemming and hawing before the important subject matter arises.

Enjoy your children during these teenage years—for all too soon they will become adults and that blessed precious time will be gone.

As every mother knows, the books on child rearing could fill entire libraries. As an herbalist and a devoted mother, I can recommend the following: *Conception, Birth and Early Childhood* by Norbert Glas, M.D., published by Anthroposophic Press in Spring Valley, New York. This is a wonderful, gentle source book of universal truths in meeting the practical problems of parenthood and gives an alternative to the usual Dr. Spock treatment. *A Child Is Born* by Wilhelm zur Linden is also available through the Anthroposophic Press. *Let's Have Healthy Children* by Adelle Davis is currently off the market because of a controversy regarding Vitamin A, but let us hope it is republished soon.

5

• • •

Herbs for Modern Beauty

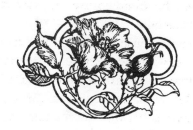

• *Hair*	• *Face*
• Shampoo	• A Mask to Clear and Smooth the Skin
• *Body*	• Simple Lotion
• Deodorant	• Simple Cream
• Bath Formulas	• Protecting Lip Gloss
• Sun Remedies	• Aftershave Lotion
• Massage and Body Oils	• Steam Treatment
• Baby or Body Powder	• Facial Soap
• Perfume	• Tooth Powder
• Treatment for Dry Hands or Feet	

We live in a complicated, difficult world full of unseen hazards in the air, water and food. These hazards often build up in our bodies causing unexplained sickness and irritations. Nowhere are possible hazards more hidden than in the cosmetics and beauty aid products that are available in any store or supermarket. Cosmetic ingredients include a veritable arsenal of hidden dangers. Compare such common ingredients as BHA or BHT, which are commonly used as preservatives to prevent oxidation of oils in cosmetics instead of a natural ingredient such as vitamin E, which works equally well. BHA and BHT are synthetic and many reports show that they can produce allergic reactions, whereas the natural vitamins show no toxicity. Thickeners such as beeswax and Candelilla wax show no toxicity when used externally, while synthetic waxes often do. Herbs such as Camomile and oils like Avocado are the most benign of substances, while their synthetic replacements can cause rather than cure irritations and blemishes.

Allergic reactions are part and parcel of commercial products. But if you make your own beauty products and medicinals *you* are in control of the contents and the products. Making your own products with simple ingredients and tested simple formulations is easy and much safer. They might not have the shelf life of the commercial products and they might not be contained in a $5 glass bottle with a 25-cent label, but they will be made of simple, natural substances that you know are harmless to your skin. Natural products can be made cleanly and with ingredients chosen especially for protection of the skin, although chronic skin problems such as acne generally mean that there is a chronic toxic condition, which no doubt has to do with improper eating or other bad habits.

The main function of the skin is to protect and to act as a defensive barrier to outside contaminants. But the skin also has a positive, healing, function. It helps to detoxify the entire body through its eliminatory capacity. The skin of the face is equipped with many sensory receptors and capillaries that allow for the healing transfer of oxygen and the elimination of wastes.

Skin care has as much to do with good nutrition, adequate rest, and plenty of exercise as it does with cosmetic preparations. If only teenagers and college girls knew this! The current fad, the "pizza pie" makeup look—green eyeshadow that looks like Green Pepper strips, round circles of glossy red on the cheeks that look like salami slices, a pale white undercoating that reminds one of melted mozzarella cheese, and Tomato-red lips—can only damage young skin and is better done without. The natural face that derives its color from exercise and the right foods with a moderate amount of coloring is more attractive and certainly healthier.

Modern girls should look at their grandmothers' clean, smooth skin and then compare it with their own lumpy blotches. Whose cosmetics are really better, the simple Cornmeal scrub and vegetable glycerine and Rosemary that grandmother applied, or the fancy scrubs with 20-syllable chemical ingredients and strange-smelling cosmetic creams and glops? The answer is simple. Homemade beauty products are the best, because the ingredients are known, the contents can be controlled, and the product can be freshly made and applied while it is still useful instead of being preserved until there is nothing left alive in it at all.

FORMULATIONS FOR THE HAIR

Shampoo. Shampoo is easy to make. And a good-quality Olive oil castile is almost as easy to make and to use. The shampoo won't be gelatinously thick, but it certainly will cleanse properly. Most shampoos contain sudsing agents as well as agents that quickly break down suds when enough water is applied. Natural shampoos don't produce copious lather but they will combine with the dirt and allow for its easy removal with a good rinse.

For 1 quart of shampoo, you will need 4 ounces of castile soap flakes and 1 quart of water or herbal infusion. Bring the water to a boil, turn off the heat, pour the water over the soap in a bowl, and stir until the soap dissolves. That's it! Add 4–8 drops of essential oil dissolved in a teaspoon of alcohol, if you like, for a pleasant scent. Start with an herbal infusion if you wish to make an herbal shampoo. The herbal infusion can be made of herbs that you have chosen and premixed for your particular type and color of hair.

HERBAL HAIR RINSE FOR NORMAL HAIR

This is a mixture of herbs that can be used as a base for the shampoo and also afterward as a rinse to both color and condition the hair, or simply as a mixture that helps to remove the soap. Mix together 1 ounce each of Camomile flowers, Marigold flowers, Comfrey leaf, and Rosemary leaf. Four ounces of mixed herbs is enough for 8 shampoos or rinses (½ ounce each use), or 4 shampoos and 4 rinses. The herbal infusion is simply made by bringing 1 quart of water to a boil and pouring this over ½ ounce (or 1 ounce if you will be using the same mixture for both shampoo and rinse) of the mixed herbs. Steep until cool enough to use. Strain carefully through a strainer or cheesecloth to remove all herb particles. If using the mixture for shampoo pour the hot herb infusion over the soap flakes until the soap dissolves. For a hair rinse pour the strained liquid over clean washed hair over and over again. The mixture need not be followed by a clear water rinse.

HERBAL HAIR RINSE FOR PROBLEM HAIR

A good mixture for problem hair or hair that is too oily or too dry is a mixture of 1 ounce each of Burdock root, Comfrey root or leaf, Rosemary leaf, and Nettle. This mixture may prove too dark for very light-colored hair. It should then be used only as the herbal infusion for the shampoo formulation above. The directions remain the same. One-half ounce of mixed herbs are infused in 1 quart of just-under-boiling water for 20 minutes or until cool enough to use, then strained and mixed with either the soap flakes or one's own shampoo, or used as a last rinse.

VINEGAR CONDITIONING HAIR RINSE

The preceding mixture of herbs can also be used as a base for an after-shampoo vinegar rinse. Apple cider vinegar is very effective to cut any soap residue that may be left over after the shampoo. It is also effective on hair that is too oily or full of dandruff, or very dark hair that needs to be conditioned. Vinegar is naturally on the acid side while a castile soap is naturally alkaline. The one balances the other and they work very effectively together. Vinegar is a solvent of oils both natural and cosmetic as well as resins. It is about 5 percent acetic acid, which is found naturally in Apples and Grapes and other foods. There is no known toxicity to vinegar. The recipe again for normal or light-colored hair is 1 ounce each of Camomile flowers, Marigold flowers, Comfrey leaf, and Rosemary leaf; and for problem hair or dark hair is 1 ounce each of Burdock root, Comfrey root, Rosemary leaf, and Nettle. Since the vinegar rinse can be stored for some time you should make enough to last for a few months. Four ounces of the mixed herbs are added to 1 quart of warm Apple cider vinegar. This is loosely capped and put away. Every day for 10–14 days the bottle is gently shaken to make sure the herbal contents stay submerged in the vinegar. At the end of this time the liquid is separated from the herbs by straining through a double layer of cheesecloth. If desired, 4–8 drops of any essential oil can be dissolved in 1 tablespoon of alcohol and added to the vinegar as a scent. This is then put into a clean bottle, labeled, and put away. When needed, up to ½ cup of the herbal vinegar is mixed with 1 cup of water and used as a last rinse after the shampoo.

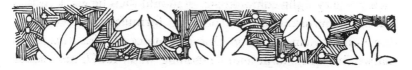

OIL TREATMENT FOR THE HAIR

Oil treatments are occasionally necessary to condition a dry scalp, a scaly scalp, sun-tortured hair, dry ends, or any type of damaged hair. They are a little more difficult to use and to apply than simple hair rinses, but a shiny, healthy head of hair may be well worth it. It is important to remember that the oil need be applied only to the scalp and not to the hair itself. Enough of the conditioning oil will drip down the hair shaft to penetrate it. The hair should first be carefully brushed to remove all loose strands of hair and grime. Wet the hair in hot water so that the oil will be more easily removed later. You can also rinse your hair in one of the hot herbal infusions as a pretreatment or steam your scalp with any of the facial steam recipes given or with the herbal rinses. Head-steaming facilitates the absorption of the oil and helps to remove any old sebaceous plugs while increasing the circulation to the scalp. The oil should be heated slightly and applied to the scalp section by section, parting the hair into sections with a rat-tail comb or pencil. After the oil is applied, wind up the hair in big hanks and secure. Wrap your head in a thin linen towel that has been dampened with any hot herbal solution, then put a plastic bag or shower cap over this, and finally a nice thick towel to hold in the heat. Leave this on for at least 30 minutes and up to 4 hours. Your head may get itchy and feel sweaty, but this is okay and only means the herbs and oil are working. Finally, remove all the wrappings and rinse the hair in hot water and then shampoo with the castile shampoo. Shampoo a second time with the juice of a Lemon added to the shampoo. Rinse again carefully and let the hair dry naturally. The hair may still feel a bit oily but this will come out when you shampoo again in a few days.

The oil treatment formulation should be a mixture of 2 ounces each of Jojoba oil, Olive oil, and Walnut oil (if possible), with ½ ounce of essential oil of Rosemary added. This 6½-ounce mixture is enough for 3–6 oil treatments that should be given no more than once every 2 weeks.

BEVERAGE TEA FOR HAIR HEALTH

It is a well-known fact that shampoo and herbal hair rinse alone will not transform drab, lanky hair into a mane of shining glory. Good nutrition and daily exercise is most important. Various nutrients are needed to keep the hair in good shape, such as cysteine (500 mg./day for at least 6 months), biotin and vitamins A, B_6, and E. Various herbs can also supply needed hair nutrients—Nettle contains absorbable iron, Horsetail contains silica, Oats and Comfrey contain calcium, and Strawberry leaves and Lemongrass contain vitamin A. A vitamin- and nutrient-supplying mixture of herbs that can be drunk as a tea is:

2	oz each of Comfrey leaf, Nettle, Lemongrass, and Violet flowers or Strawberry leaves
1	ounce each of Kelp or Dulse, Beet tops, Alfalfa, and Lemon peel
1/2	oz each of Hibiscus flowers, Camomile, Oatstraw, Horsetail, and Mint

These herbs are mixed and bottled in a dry, lightproof container and stored. The tea is brewed in the usual way, 1 teaspoon to 1 tablespoon of herbs to 1 cup of boiling water, steeped, strained, and drunk. Honey can be added if desired. For best results the tea should be taken regularly over some period of time, 2–4 cups per day.

SETTING LOTION

Easy-to-use natural hair-setting lotions can be made with any of the gums or the seaweeds. Irish moss is especially easy to use. One-quarter ounce is boiled with 1 quart of water for 20 minutes until it is thick and gooey. This is strained through a coarse strainer into a squatty wide-mouth glass jar. Add 2 tablespoons of alcohol, or for scent add an essential oil that has been dissolved in the alcohol. You can use 2 tablespoons of Bay rum, which is alcohol-based. You can also start with any herbal infusion instead of plain water to get the benefits of the herbs. Rosemary water is especially good, as is Lemongrass water. This formula would then be ½ ounce Irish moss and ½ ounce Rosemary or Lemongrass boiled in 1 quart of water until thick. To use the lotion simply dip your comb into it, comb through the hair, and roll up the hair in the usual way.

DRY SHAMPOO

Dry shampoos are normally used during cold weather to strip the hair of grime and grease and excess oils without wetting the hair, which may cause the person to get chilled and catch cold. They are also useful as a conditioner for limp, greasy hair. My favorite dry shampoo is a mixture of 1 part each of finely ground Cornmeal, Almonds finely ground, and powdered Orris root. One tablespoon of each, mixed, should be more than adequate for a single shampoo. First the hair is brushed and brushed, then the mixture is rubbed into the scalp. The hair is brushed again. Some of the particles may be left in the hair, but this is okay. Leave them in until the next time you intend to wet shampoo, then brush the hair, shampoo, and treat as usual. Your hair will have an unusual luster and gloss not to be had by any other means.

CONDITIONING OIL

The finest mixture of conditioning oils is Jojoba, Rosemary, and Basil. Equal parts of the oils are mixed, and 1 drop is used at a time. Put the conditioning oil on your hand, rub your hand across your brush, and then brush your hair. Remember to bend at the waist to release tension from the neck and shoulder muscles and brush from the nape of the neck all the way down to the ends of the hair. One or 2 drops of oil on the brush is more than adequate for your daily ritual.

FORMULATIONS FOR THE BODY

Deodorant. Deodorants come in all forms, from a simple application of baking soda or white clay that absorbs moistures and odor to the chemical formulas that prevent perspiration. These latter can be harmful, as they actually stop the body from "breathing" through the skin. But they can be useful when you have beautiful clothing that you don't wish to get stained. Homemade deodorants do two things: They minimize odor and they absorb wetness. Some herbs that have a deodorant action (something that destroys or masks unpleasant odors) do stain garments, although this shouldn't happen with deodorants made with clay or baking soda. Normally, simply washing the underarms or the feet several times a day and being scrupulous about the cleanliness of your underclothes and socks is all that is necessary to keep body smells away. Naturally a diet rich in vegetables and whole grains and vitamin supplements like zinc and vitamin C is also necessary to keep you sweet-smelling from the inside out.

DEODORANT FORMULA 1

Mix equal quantities of baking soda and white clay, put into an old-fashioned dusting powder box, and dust on with a puff whenever necessary.

DEODORANT FORMULA 2

Mix 2 tablespoons each of baking soda and white clay and add 1 tablespoon of powdered Lemon peel or Orange peel as a scent.

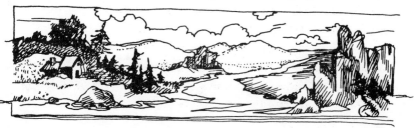

DEODORANT TEA

Mix Sage leaves, Sagebrush, Melilot, Parsley, and Alfalfa in equal quantities. Store the mixture in a lightproof container. Drink ½ cup of tea 4 times per day regularly. Brew the tea in the usual way.

Bath Formulas. Mixtures of herbs that are effective in treating various skin conditions, or that smooth, sooth, and hydrate the skin, are easily obtained from herb or health food stores. They are also easy to make and economical. Bath herbs are the organic antidote to impure air conditions and harsh chlorinated water.

The herbs themselves can be placed directly in the bathtub, although this may lead to a stopped-up drain. They can also be wrapped in a washcloth, secured with a rubber band, and used as a scrub cloth. Small cheesecloth or muslin bags can be purchased or made, the herbal mixtures inserted within, and the entire bag thrown into the tub, where it can release the essence of its herbal contents. My favorite method of taking an herb bath is to make a standard herbal infusion of 1 ounce mixed herbs steeped in 1 quart of very hot water for 20 minutes, the entire contents then strained directly into the warm bath water, and the herbs themselves wrapped and tied in a washcloth, which is used to scrub the body after a soak in the bath.

Skin conditioners can also be made from simple household ingredients like Cornmeal, Oatmeal, Almond meal, and salt. These are used separately or mixed in any amounts. A small handful is scrubbed on the body, which removes old dead skin, softening the skin and conditioning it, making it smooth and soft. Then a bath or shower is taken, and this constitutes an entire beauty ritual.

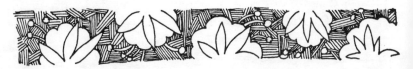

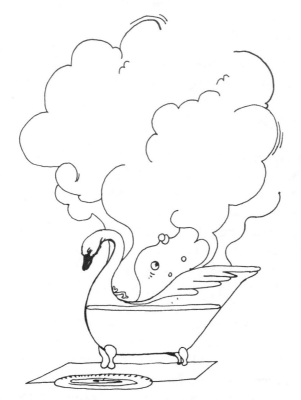

BATH FORMULA FOR DRY SKIN

1   oz Oatmeal
1   oz Almond meal
1   oz ground Comfrey leaves

Mix ingredients. This mixture is enough for 4 baths or showers. One ounce of the mixture is simmered for 20 minutes over
low heat with 1 quart of water. This should be poured through
a strainer into the tub. What is left in the strainer is used as a
scrub for the entire body. To scrub, take small handfuls and
simply scrub directly on the skin. When you finally get into the
tub and begin your soak you will certainly feel smooth and
relaxed. The herbal liquid that will have gone through the
strainer and into the bath water will complete the smoothing
and hydrating (moisture adding) process.

BATH FORMULA FOR OILY OR SCALY SKIN

1   oz Lemongrass herb
1   oz Cornmeal
1   oz Witch Hazel herb
1   oz Rose petals

Mix these ingredients. One ounce of the mixed herbs is enough for 1 bath or shower. Add it to 1 quart of boiling water. Turn off the heat and let steep for 20 minutes. Strain the mixture through a strainer directly into the bath and use the residue as a direct scrub to the skin. Step into the bath and soak for at least 10 minutes, wash, and dry off. Use this mixture at least twice a week.

BATH OIL

A good bath oil may be made using 4 ounces of oil, 1 ounce of Ivory liquid soap, and ¼ ounce of essential oil. Bath oils are best made with fruit kernel oils plus Wheat germ oil. They are concentrated, and only an ounce is added to the bath. A good combination would be 1 ounce each of Wheat germ oil, Sesame oil, Olive oil, and Almond oil. The Ivory liquid soap, mixed with the oils, allows the mixture to disperse somewhat in the bath water. Use whatever essential oil pleases you. Mint oils are stimulating, Sage oil is useful for tired muscles, Rose and Jasmine oils are very relaxing, Lavender is cleansing and mildly stimulating, and Sandalwood is relaxing.

Sun remedies. Lemon juice put on the skin hastens a tan, plain mayonnaise is a sun protectant, PABA is a vitamin that actually blocks the harmful rays, and vitamin E nourishes the skin and keeps it from burning. These can be mixed in various ways to protect the skin and to encourage good color. My favorite application to lubricate sun-soaked skin is simply pure Corn oil that I slather on every few hours.

SUNTAN LOTION

In a blender mix together 2 ounces of rich saltless mayonnaise (preferably the homemade type made with Olive oil and Lemon juice), 2 ounces of very dark black tea, and the juice of 1 Lemon. Pour this into a container and squeeze into it the contents of five 400-IU capsules of vitamin E oil. Use this regularly, before and after swimming, to encourage a good tan.

SUNBURN LOTION

If you should get a nasty burn, the simple application of something cold will help to cool the skin. This can be a cool bath until the skin cools, the juice of the Aloe plant, or simply a compress of Apple cider vinegar. If you have the Aloe gel in a bottle, make continual applications of this until the skin cools. Direct application of vitamin E oil is also extremely useful to cool and heal burned skin. Liquid vitamin C plus Aloe Vera juice and gel is a super healer for a bad sunburn, or for that matter any sort of a burn.

Massage and Body Oils. Massage and body oils are mixtures of oils and possibly herbal extracts that by their application are relaxing, healing, soothing, or stimulating; they can be scented or not; they can be used as a medium to hold medicinal herbs, or they can simply be creamy mixtures that you apply after the bath or after a day in the sun. Massage and body oils can be oily or watery, depending on ingredients—they can even be thick like a cream. They are best applied in small amounts and rubbed carefully into theh face or body, or small amounts can be added to the bath for dry skin. They can be a medium to absorb essential oils or vitamin oils.

MASSAGE OIL

To make a basic massage oil, bring 1 quart of mixed oils and 1 ounce of mixed herbs to a gentle boil. Using a nonmetal pot and a very low heat, gently simmer for about 20 minutes, then remove the pot from the flame and allow the mixture to cool. Then strain the herbal oil through a double layer of cheesecloth, bottle, label, add a scent if you wish, and the mixture is ready for use.

The oil can be a combination that contains all the essential fatty acids (such as Corn, Safflower, Soy, Olive, and Peanut), or it can be simply Olive oil or a mixture of fruit and nut oils such as Apricot kernel, Almond, Avocado, or Walnut. Herbs: For dry skin, use Alfalfa, Rose, and Camomile; for oily skin, use Lemongrass, Witch Hazel, and Marigold; to stimulate, use Peppermint, Rosemary, and Thyme; to relax, use Sage, Catnip, and Camomile. The essential oil may be chosen to enhance the effect of the herbs or simply to please your senses.

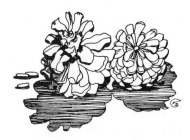

Bath or Body Powder. Body powders can be made of mixtures of baking soda, Cornstarch, Rice powder, Oatmeal powder, herbs, and talcum. They can be used to cure heat rash or chafing, or simply to absorb moisture and provide "slip" so that clothing can be easily put on and taken off. Most of these materials come in a powdered form, but if they don't it is a simple matter to run your materials through a seed grinder or Coffee mill to create a soft powder. Oatmeal and herbs are very healing and can be used for diaper rash or any sort of skin irritation.

BABY POWDER

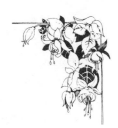

1	oz Camomile flowers
1	oz Marigold flowers
1	oz Oats or Oatmeal
1/2	oz Comfrey root
1/2	oz eggshells

These should be purchased in the finest form possible and then put through a seed grinder or Coffee mill until they have been ground very fine. Sift the entire contents through a fine sifter and bottle. What doesn't make it through the sifter should be discarded. For babies, especially if heat rash is a problem, add about ½ ounce Cornstarch.

BODY POWDER

1	oz plain talcum
1	oz crushed and sifted eggshells
1/2	oz powdered Sandalwood

Mix and dust on the body whenever desired.

PLAIN BODY POWDER

1	oz plain talcum
1	oz crushed and sifted eggshells
4	drops essential oil

Mix these ingredients, except for the essential oil. Drop the oil over the powder and stir with a fork. Let it sit for a few days and then sift and resift 5 or 6 times through a regular flour sifter. This will nicely distribute the essential oil throughout the entire mixture. Let it sit again for a few days until the oil can completely vaporize and mix with the other ingredients. Dust on the body after the bath.

Perfume. Making your own perfume can be as simple as dissolving an essential oil that you like in pure alcohol and water and using it as a cologne or toilet water. It can also be as complicated as picking your own flowers and extracting their scent through various semicomplicated processes. Commercial perfumes and colognes made from real flowers cost many, many dollars. Granted they come in very attractive containers with designer labels, but after all, it is the contents that count. Walk out into your own garden or into an herb store and smell the fragrance. You can easily make fragrances that please you and work with your own body chemistry. Perfumes and toilet waters are not that difficult to make, and the contents can be controlled so that the fragrance you wear is really something you like.

MACERATION TECHNIQUE

To macerate means to extract and soften by soaking in a fluid. Pick fresh flowers and remove all the green parts. Put the flowers in a container and add just enough Olive oil to barely cover the flowers. As the flowers soak up the oil they will sink deeper into the oil. You need just the thinnest layer of oil over the flowers to extract the essence. Within 24 hours most flowers will have given up their essential oil to the surrounding oil medium. The flowers are now dead and can be removed by careful straining. Smell the oil—if it has retained the fragrance of the flowers that you started with, you have a perfume oil. If not, then add fresh flowers to the oil and repeat the process. When your oil finally smells like flowers and not like olive oil you are through. This oil can be preserved by the addition of tincture of Benzoin, a natural preservative that occurs as a resin in a tree and is available in most pharmacies. Add 4 drops of tincture of Benzoin for every ounce of perfume oil.

Treatment for Dry Hands or Feet. Sometimes when we have done dishes by hand for a number of years or because of the type of work we do, our hands can get very dry, cracked, painful, and unsightly. The continual application of a healing oil is helpful but there are other emergency measures that can be very effective. Once a woman called me and told me that her hands had been cracked and bleeding for 3 years and she hadn't been able to adequately do the housework or the dishes. My first suggestion was that she cut down on the amount of housework that she was doing and wear rubber gloves. She had apparently become allergic to household cleansers and dishwashing liquids. Her doctor had suggested these same things and in addition had prescribed a medication that had not been helpful. My second suggestion was to use a 300-year-old remedy that is called in the old receipt books, "To Whiten and Smooth the Hands." This totally cured and healed this woman's painful, cracked hands within days. It is very simple, although slightly messy to make and use.

SOFT HANDS FORMULA

1   oz ground Almonds
1   beaten egg
1/4   oz ground Comfrey root

Mix all the ingredients, add 1 tablespoon of honey, and mix it with your hands. Carefully coat your hands from wrist to fingernails. Ask someone to help you put on a pair of kid gloves over the entire mess. (You can use cotton gloves, but the stuff will leak out through the night and make a mess on the bed, so it is best to use kid gloves.) And go to bed. In the morning, remove and rinse the gloves and rinse your hands. Apply any of the lotions or creams described below. Repeat this process every night for a week, then once a week for a month, and then once a month for as long as necessary. This is a very effective measure for sore hands or feet.

FORMULATIONS FOR THE FACE

A Mask to Clear and Smooth the Skin. Masks can remove grime or old, dead skin, improve circulation, treat and heal pimples, remove excess oil and hydrate dry skin, nourish, texturize, and smooth. Again, they are so simple and easy to make, so economical that it seems foolish to spend $6 or $8 for a 4-ounce jar in a store. The best ingredients for masks are egg white, honey, any mashed fruit, brewer's yeast, cooked Oatmeal, or clay. Any of these can be used singly or in combination. Egg white is refining, clay can remove pimples and grime, brewer's yeast is extremely powerful as a circulation stimulant, and honey is naturally acid–balanced and can balance either an oily or a dry complexion. Simply wash your face, pat it dry, apply a mask, let it dry, and rinse it off. If necessary apply a lotion to prevent dryness. Use a mask regularly, but no more than 3 times a week.

REFRESHING MINT SOUFFLÉ

1	T ground or powdered Spearmint
1	T honey
1	T oil

Mix in a blender until nice and fluffy and apply to clean skin.

OILY SKIN MASK

| 1 | T clay |
| 1 | T water or Lemon juice |

Mix in the palm of your hand and apply to clean skin.

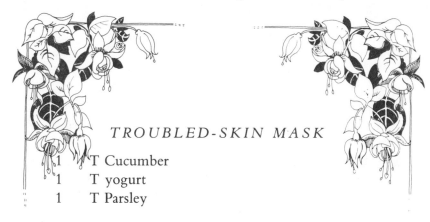

TROUBLED-SKIN MASK

1   T Cucumber
1   T yogurt
1   T Parsley

Blend in a blender until fluffy, apply to clean skin.

Simple Lotion. Lotions are used for oily skin, contain more water than they do oils, and can be used for the entire body or complexion. They can soften lines that are beginning to form or remove excess oil. A very basic lotion is the one Grandmother made from vegetable glycerin and Rosewater. Rosewater is made at home by gently simmering Rose petals in water for 10 minutes, straining, and preserving with a bit of alcohol or simply refrigerating. Fine-quality Rosewater can be purchased in liquor stores or Middle Eastern groceries, and also in herb and health food stores. Lotions can be applied any time from morning until night, but should only be applied to clean skin. Remember that herbal mixtures should be used as soon as possible, as bacteria can build up in lotions and creams when they do not contain preservatives. About 3 days in the fridge should be the limit before they are thrown out.

ROSE AND ROSEMARY LOTION

1   oz Rosemary tea
1   oz Rose petal tea or Rosewater
1   T egg white

Mix in a blender and keep refrigerated.

ORANGE LOTION

1/2	oz melted Cocoa butter
1	oz warm Olive oil
1	oz Orange juice
2	drops essential oil (Orange flavor if possible)

Mix all these ingredients in a blender until light and fluffy; bottle, label, and use. This need not be refrigerated but it should be used as soon as possible. It may separate but can be beaten together again with a small spoon.

Simple Cream. Creams are more oily than lotions and are more suitable as nighttime applications or for dry skin. They are used as skin softeners, to moisturize, or to nourish by providing essential vitamins, or they can simply be used as "cleansing" creams. The simplest and least expensive is any type of supermarket shortening with the addition of herb waters or vitamins. Crisco plus vitamin E oil is excellent as a nighttime moisturizer. Crisco by itself is useful to remove daytime makeup. Mayonnaise is an excellent cream as long as it is made with Olive oil and Lemon juice rather than oil and vinegar. The egg in the mayonnaise is extremely nourishing to dry skin. A good basic formula combines 1 ounce of beeswax, 3 ounces of oil, a bit of scent, and a tablespoon or two of herb water. These are all heated gently, removed from the heat, whipped until cool with a whisk, bottled, labeled, and used.

REJUVENATING CREAM

1	oz beeswax or lanolin
3	oz Almond oil
1	ampule of Elastin or 4 vitamin E capsules
2	drops oil of Rose

Follow the basic directions.

STIMULATING CREAM

1   oz beeswax or lanolin
3   oz Wheat germ oil
1   oz strong Peppermint tea
1   drop oil of Peppermint

Follow the basic directions.

Protecting Lip Gloss. Lip glosses are used to protect the lips and to add color. Lip gloss can also be used on the cheeks or the chin for color. Lip glosses are highly protective for swimmers or skiers to protect the delicate lip tissue from overexposure to the sun and elements.

BASIC LIP GLOSS

2   t melted beeswax
4   T colored Sesame oil (for color you must first soak the plant Alkanet in Sesame oil for 2 weeks: The oil, now dark red, is strained and used)
1   dab Camphor (for chapped lips) or Menthol (for minty taste) or ½ dab each

Put these ingredients together in a very small pot and heat them until almost melted. Remove from the heat, beat until cool, put up in a small container, and continue to whip until cold or set.

Aftershave Lotion. Men can use all the previous formulas but in addition they need an astringent lotion or something that can be used after they shave to soothe the irritated flesh.

Witch Hazel extract is a simple standard herbal remedy to use as an aftershave lotion. It is cheap and easily available. It can be mixed in any amount with Rosewater to make a more pleasantly scented soothing lotion. A more soothing lotion can be made by boiling 1 tablespoon of Quince seeds in 1 cup of water until a gel forms. The gel is then diluted with an herb water, such as Rose or Orange water, to whatever consistency you like and then used. This should be made in small amounts so that it can be used before it spoils.

Another simple aftershave formulation is an equal mixture of plain vegetable glycerin and any herb water. Comfrey tea is useful for irritated skin, Bay rum (purchase in a pharmacy) "closes" the pores, Mint tea is stimulating, and Rose or Jasmine flower water is soothing and nicely scented.

Another nice mixture is Apple cider vinegar mixed equally with glycerin or Witch hazel extract. The Apple cider vinegar can have had herbs infused in it that have been strained. Even the vinegar conditioning rinses previously described can be used as a base for this aftershave lotion.

Steam Treatment. Clear, beautiful skin is ultimately the result of good nutrition and regular exercise. Nutritional supplements help, as do pure wholesome substances that are used on the skin. But in dire conditions (for example, where there is a lot of air pollution) or for a special occasion when you want your skin really pore-deep clean, nothing beats a steam treatment. A

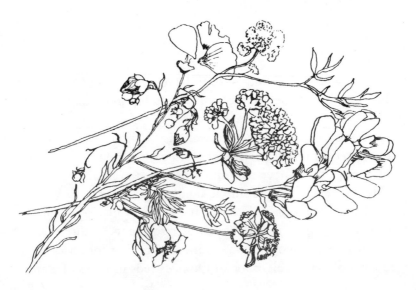

steam bath is a steam treatment for the entire body, but steam can be used as a treatment for the face or scalp as regularly as you boil water or use a vaporizer in your bedroom.

For skin steaming you need a pot, some water, some herbs, and a towel. Bring 1 quart of water and about ½ ounce of herbs to a boil in the pot. Put the steaming pot on the table and put your face over the pot but not less than 10 inches from the water. Cover the head and pot with the towel and relax for at least 5 minutes. The boiling water releases the aromatic and healing essence of the herbs and the volatile oils, which are then absorbed into the skin to do their magic work. Naturally, the steaming increases circulation and perspiration, which cleans the pores from the inside out. This is very refreshing and adds moisture to moisture-starved skin. Steaming with the right herbs can also relieve tension and unclog stuffy sinuses.

BASIC FORMULATIONS

Use 1 tablespoon each of any herbs that you may have available, but especially Licorice, Fennel seed, Mint leaves, Comfrey leaves, and Parsley. Other herbs can be added, such as flowers and scented leaves, but these herbs should form the basic recipe.

Facial Soap. Normally soap is alkaline, the skin slightly acid. The alkaline suds dissolve the dirt, combine with it, so that it can be washed off. The skin returns to its normal acid condition within minutes of being washed. For many people alkaline soap seems too strong and drying to use on the face. In this case some of the "acid-balanced" soaps or gentle soaps such as Neca-7 or Sinalca can be used.

You can also "gentle" your own favorite bar soap by simply chopping it up in a small pot and melting it with a dab of honey and 1 ounce of herb water. The herb water can be Camomile or Lettuce for soothing the skin, Lavender for stimulation and removing excess oils, Rose water for toning, or Comfrey for healing.

Tooth Powder. Beautiful teeth are an asset to any person and these too can be taken care of at home with simple home remedies. Brush regularly with a soft brush, floss at least once a day, and start your day by eating a crisp Apple. Many people recommend tongue and teeth brushing in the morning, but eating an Apple does the same thing and is infinitely more preferable and pleasant.

Easy tooth powders include the well-known combination of baking soda and table salt. Kelp can be substituted for the salt and various powdered herbs can be added for flavor. For scent add 1 drop of essential oil to every ounce of salt and soda. Stir the mixture and let it sit so that the salt and soda can absorb the scent. Press this through a strainer, bottle, and label. Cinnamon oil is good as a scent, Myrrh oil is especially recommended as an antiseptic aromatic, and Wintergreen or Birch can be added for a minty taste, while Rosemary or Basil or both can be added to improve circulation.

A SPECIAL DAY

Summer is that beautiful golden time of year when we acquire our summer skin with its rich, warm, rosy glow, but it can also be a time of dry skin characterized by scaly legs and arms, skin so suntanned it looks gray, and hair that is dry and dull. The remedy for all these sun excesses is to reserve 1 day a month, especially in the summer, as a "Take Care of Yourself Day." This is important for the external health of both men and women. Your day a month should probably be on a weekend when you will not have to go to work or school. Maybe you can charm a grandparent or friend into having the children for the day. There is nothing worse than to be surrounded in the bathtub by a flock of children laughing at Mommy, who is covered with a blue clay mask and wrapped in strands of herbs from nose to toes, or at Daddy with egg in his hair and beard and Wheat germ oil on his face and chest.

Step 1: Hands. The night before your special day, make a mush of egg-honey-ground Almonds (Almond meal) and powdered Comfrey root, about a teaspoon of each, and cover your hands with it. Then either wrap your hands in plastic bags tied at the wrist with string or pull on a pair of large kid or leather gloves. This treatment softens the skin and heals any nicks or cuts while restoring detergent- or work-roughened dry hands.

Step 2: Internal Flushing. Drink plenty of herbal teas (DetoxTea or the mixture listed in Step 4), 1–3 quarts, throughout the day to cleanse the inner body.

Step 3: Hair. In the morning after a wonderful refreshing sleep, wash the paste off your hand and prepare an oil treatment for your dry sunblown hair. Mix either 4 tablespoons of pure saltless mayonnaise or 2 ounces of Olive oil with ¼ ounce of pure essential oil of Rosemary. Warm this mixture in a water bath or double boiler. Wet your hair to keep the Rosemary oil and mayonnaise or Rosemary oil and Olive oil off the hair, and apply this mixture to the hair roots and hair ends only. You will probably want to continuously part your hair with a rat-tail comb so that the oil will only get on the scalp. If you and a friend are doing the day together, you can work on each other, which will make the parting and applying easier. It is especially helpful for you and your husband or male friend to do this together so you can have someone to laugh with; laughing relieves stress and adds beauty while subtracting lines from the face. After completely oiling and massaging your scalp, cover your hair with a muslin bag about 18 inches square that is filled with 2 ounces of hot, moistened herbs. You can use the same combination of herbs that you will use for the facial steaming. Cover the muslin bag with a plastic bag to keep in the heat and then cover with a towel.

Step 4: Face (Steaming). Make a mixture of herbs, such as Camomile, Comfrey, Peppermint, and Lavender. Put a handful of this mixture into a muslin bag and put it into a pot with a quart of water. Bring the mixture to a boil, transfer the pot to a table, and let the steam play on your face for at least 5 minutes. If you are fortunate enough to have a hot tub, put bags of this mixture into the hot tub for your face and body. A steam or sauna is also appropriate, because it heats those herbs that are on your head, which continues the treatment of the scalp while the herb on the face clears and cleanses the face.

Step 5: Face and Eyes (Cleansing). Make a mixture of clay and herbs. The color of the clay depends on the condition of the skin. Blue and white clay are for dry or sensitive skin, red clay for oily skin, green clay for any type skin, and the dark or black clays for drawing out impurities or blackheads. (I used blue clay for the dry areas and red clay for the oily areas.) Mix 2 tablespoons clay, 2 teaspoons sea salt, 1 teaspoon granular Kelp, 1 teaspoon powdered Comfrey or Ginseng, and 1 teaspoon honey melted in 3 tablespoons of hot water or some of the hot herbal water from Step 3. The mixture will be thick but creamy. Apply it generously to your face or to any part of your body that needs cleansing and firming. Rub it on in circular motions to gently sand the skin. Now lie down for 20 minutes on a slant board with herb tea bags on your eyes (such as Camomile, Fennel, or Parsley for brightening and reducing bags under the eyes). This treatment cleanses the face, peels waxy dead, dull skin by the mild sanding action of the salt and Kelp, and texturizes and firms sagging skin as the clay and honey dries. Of course, you still have the plastic bag covering the muslin herb bag and towel on your probably by now sweaty head.

Step 6: Body and Shampoo. Now is the time to jump directly into a hot, relaxing bath. Add the pot of water with the facial herbs as well as the muslin bag on your head to the bath water. Relax in the tub for 20–30 minutes or more. Scrub your skin all over with a loofah and then with the muslin bags of herbs. Scrub off the facial mask gently with a washcloth using a circular up and out motion. Soak your head to loosen the mayonnaise or oil and then shampoo with a gentle herbal shampoo.

Step 7: Rinsing and Toning. After you are thoroughly relaxed and scrubbed, let the water run out of the tub, stand up, and take a long hot and then warm shower, thoroughly rinsing your hair. Apply your favorite hair conditioner and rinse. Take a 2-minute cold shower, then step out with your renewed body and tone your face and body. A skin toner freshens and tightens the pores, enlivening the skin. Use a mixture of Lemon juice and Mint water for oily skin, plain old-fashioned Rosewater and glycerin for normal skin, and Orange flower water and glycerin for dry or sensitive skin. Always tone your skin moving your hands gently from the center outward and from bottom to top. Start skin toning with a lotion and a massage that starts under the jaw and works up to the hair line. The flower waters are available in any liquor store or body-care center, while the glycerin can be purchased at an pharmacy.

Now that you are clean from head to toe, inside and out, relaxed and refreshed, you still have the rest of the day to lie back in an easy chair and read or to do a little gardening, or even to take a nap. You might also exchange massages with a partner using an herbal body oil. I guarantee that you will feel like a 100 percent new person who has exchanged that dry old dull skin for a bright and shiny new one.

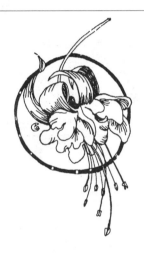

6

. . .

Dieting and Fasting

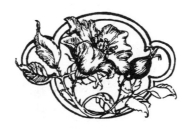

So you woke up this morning, bent over to tie your shoe, and realized that in order to do this you had to push your tummy bulge out of the way and bring your foot up to your hands instead of bringing your hands down to your foot. What does this mean? It means, my friend, that you have to lose weight. Somewhere along the way, probably slowly, flab crept up on you. Maybe flesh was added to your body at the rate of 1 pound per month. In a year, without noticing, you had gained 12 pounds. So what can you do about it? There are two simple rules for losing weight: Eat less and exercise more. If this sounds easy, it is . . . and it isn't. You need to moderate your habits and exercise will power when it comes to food.

Eat less. Eat half as much as you normally do and use a smaller plate. Little tricks help, like those mentioned in my *Herbal Guide to Inner Health;* take smaller portions and always leave a few bites on the plate (in direct opposition to your mum, who said, "Eat everything on your plate, dear, remember the starving kids in ———!"). These tricks concentrate your attention on the amount of food you normally consume, helping you consume less.

Exercise more. This means all the usual things like walking up the stairs instead of taking the elevator, walking to the grocery store rather than driving, trying to follow your kids, movement for movement, leap for leap, rather than sitting on the bench and watching them play. Most of all it means setting aside a period during the day, every day, to exercise in a concentrated manner for at least 20 minutes. It doesn't matter whether you run, jog, swim, roller skate, play tennis or volleyball, or practice yoga—anything that makes you move your body with control and vigor is essential.

So that's it. *Eat less and exercise more.*

But you are probably asking what part herbs play in losing weight. All the toxins and poisons that we accumulate (by breathing, eating, drinking) and absorb are stored in the fat. During the dieting process, the fat in the body is used for energy and the toxins are eventually liquefied and released via the bloodstream through the various excretory processes. Sweating, urinating, and defecating are the body's releasing mechanisms. DDT is one of the toxins, and there are many more. As the fat is liquefied into the bloodstream it releases the toxins and they, in effect, poison us. This is called autointoxification. These poisons are what cause the queasy sick feelings during a prolonged fast or diet. When we take herbs, they help in the detoxification process and protect us from feeling sick. They are also foods, providing nutrients, vitamins, and minerals that help replenish the body's store of these substances.

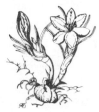

DIET AND FASTING HERBS

Alfalfa herb and sprouts *(Medicago sativa)* should be drunk as a tea or eaten throughout any diet or fast. Alfalfa is loaded with vitamins, minerals, protein, and contains enzymes that help in the digestive process. It also has an oxidizing effect on the blood. Taken cold, the tea is an excellent diuretic and a mild aperient (a mild stimulant for the bowels). Drunk hot and mixed with Pennyroyal and Catnip, the tea acts as a diaphoretic, reducing fever and thereby helping the cleansing or detoxification of the body through sweating. Alfalfa also seems to stimulate the growth of the connective tissues.

BLACKBERRY LEAVES (Rubus fruticosus) are a valuable astringent, considered an effective "blood cleanser," useful in improving blood circulation. Eat the ripe fruit to correct diarrhea. Gather and dry young shoots or canes of the Blackberry and use them in tea mixtures for curbing diarrhea, as a gargle for throat inflammations, or in douching formulations to clear up any sort of vaginal discharge.

CAMOMILE (Anthemis nobilus and Matricaria chamomilla) is an herb whose flower is drunk as a tea. It has a powerful alkalinizing effect on the blood as well as being a digestive and nervine. Camomile is antispasmodic, soothing, and slightly sedating—an excellent addition to the reducing diet, as its main function is to detoxify and soothe the entire system.

CELERY (Apium graveolens) has a cleansing, diuretic effect. It is drunk as a tea or juiced with other herbs to be used as a healing, alkalinizing tonic to the system. Fresh Celery can be juiced and is considered to be a solvent of uric acid, which makes it very helpful in treating rheumatism or arthritis. Whether eaten or drunk it has a calming effect on the nerves.

CHERRY STEMS (Prunus avium and other species), *Corn silk* (flower pistils of *Zea Mays*) and Couchgrass (*Agropyron* or *Triticum repens*) are all healing, astringent tonics that act on the urinary system. They have a diuretic effect and are used in all problems of the kidneys and bladder, especially when both a demulcent and a diuretic effect are needed.

Comfrey (Symphytum officinale) is an ancient healing herb known to the Greeks and Romans. It is healing, a soothing emollient and a demulcent. One of the few plant sources of B_{12}, it is also high in calcium and is a cellular regenerative.

Dandelion (Taraxacum officinale) is a specific for the liver. Beneficial for anyone who suffers from an excess of uric acid, like Celery it is food for the rheumatic and the arthritic. Dandelions are extremely rich in vitamins C and A as well as mineral salts. The roots can be roasted and ground and used as a healthful substitute for Coffee.

Dulse and other seaweeds are extremely useful in any fasting or detoxifying diet. Sea plants contain all the vitamins and minerals needed in the diet. The algin in sea plants combines with toxic elements in the body, enabling us to excrete these elements harmlessly. Also, the large amounts of iodine in seaweeds stimulate the thyroid gland.

Elder (Sambucus nigra) leaves and flowers have an astringent action, the roots a diuretic one. The leaves and roots are both useful for inflammations. Taken hot, the tea acts as an intense diaphoretic, reducing fever and cleansing the body via the sweat glands.

Fennel (Foeniculum vulgare) roots and seeds are carminative, stimulative, and diuretic. They help the body to detoxify through the various excretory functions. A standard slimming herb, it also contains substances that are similar to human hormones, a property useful for both men and women. It is said that the ancient Greeks gave Fennel to their Olympic competitors to increase strength while preventing weight gain.

Lemon juice and Lemon peel (Citrus Limon) is an alkalinizing substance that contains vitamin C and bioflavonoids. Lemons benefit all systems of the body and are especially useful mixed with Dandelion herb to heal the liver. During fasting an excellent liver tonic is obtained by mixing 3 tablespoons Olive oil with the juice of 2 Lemons, some grated Ginger root, and the juice of 1 Grapefruit. Drink this down with 3–5 crushed cloves of Garlic. For 10 days, drink this mixture early every morning, drink only Obesi-Tea or Detox-Tea (recipes follow) and eat only steamed vegetables. This 10-day cleansing diet will detoxify the body and heal the digestive system.

Mint (Mentha genus) is useful in fasting and dieting as it is deliciously aromatic. Adding mint to any tea will give it a pleasant and tangy flavor.

Parsley (Petroselinum crispum) is a rich source of vitamins and minerals. It is extremely important in weight loss diets. Parsley is stimulating and is recommended for jaundice, the liver and the kidneys, cellulite, and arthritis. Always add Parsley to vegetable juices to increase their efficacy.

HERBAL RECIPES

These herbs are all foods as well as medicines. They should become part of the reducing diet, especially in the form of tea, for their detoxifying quality. Several formulas work extremely well.

The dried, cut herbs should be mixed and stored. You can use fresh herbs but naturally they cannot be mixed in advance. Whatever is fresh can also be mixed with dried herbs, but added just before brewing.

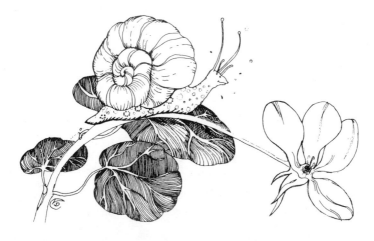

DETOX-TEA

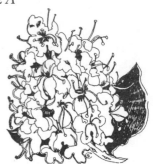

2	oz Celery tops and seeds
1	oz Fennel seeds
2	oz Parsley
2	oz Corn Silk
1	oz Cherry stems
2	oz Dandelion
2	oz Couchgrass
4	oz Blackberry leaves

Mix these herbs and store in a jar. This amount should last for 1 month. Take ½ ounce of the mixed herbs and pour over them 2–4 cups of boiling water. Steep overnight and drink the entire 2–4 cups of tea, cold, in small sips throughout the next day.

OBESI-TEA

2	oz Mint
2	oz Dandelion
2	oz Celery tops
1	oz Lemon peel
2	oz Camomile
2	oz Parsley
2	oz Alfalfa
2	oz Comfrey leaf
2	oz Dulse
1	oz Elder flower and leaf
2	oz Fennel seed

Use same method as for Detox-Tea.

FASTING

Begin a 10-day fast by resting and relaxing the system with simple foods such as grains, vegetables, and salads. For 2–3

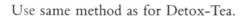

days eat only slightly steamed vegetables and sip vegetable juice. Then stop eating altogether and drink only 2–4 quarts of liquid (water or herb tea or both) every day for 8 days. Use Detox-Tea or Obesi-Tea or both. Vitamin and mineral supplements are necessary, especially vitamin C, taken at the rate of 2–5 grams per day. You can purchase a useful stress formula containing B vitamins and minerals at any health food store. Because it is important to satisfy the chewing needs of the body, start or end the day by slowly eating and savoring every morsel of 1 crunchy Apple. Chewing an Apple is essential for the health of your teeth and easy elimination. At the end of 10 days resume eating, but only steamed vegetables, vegetable and Lettuce salads, and vegetable juices. For the first 4 days, eat frequently but keep the portions small. Then resume your normal diet; that is, vegetables and grains at supper, protein or nuts and seeds for lunch, and fruits for breakfast (maybe some yogurt too). The normal diet should be an alkaline one.

ALKALINE FOODS

An alkaline diet is an effective nutritional aid, which helps balance the physical and mental functions that have been thrown into disharmony by poor health and eating habits. This simply means eating foods that provide an abundance of alkaline elements. When foods are eaten they are oxidized, which leads to the formation of a residue or ash. If this residue contains the minerals sodium, potassium, calcium, and magnesium, the foods are designated alkaline ash foods. If the residue is predominantly sulfur, phosphorus, chlorine, and uncombusted organic acid radicals the foods are designated acid ash foods. Dried Figs are the most alkaline while Rye grain is the most acidic.

The entire eliminative system of the body is strengthened and the nervous system relaxed by alkaline foods. The body seems to function best when 70–80 percent of the diet is composed of alkaline foods.

ALKALINE (AL) AND ACIDIC (ac) FOODS

PROTEIN

Soybeans	AL
Raw milk, nonfat	AL
Buttermilk	ac
Cottage cheese	ac
Yogurt	ac
Eggs	ac
Cheeses	ac
Yeast	ac
Raw milk, whole	ac
Fish	ac
Fowl	ac
Meat of any sort	ac

VEGETABLES

Asparagus	ac
Artichoke	ac
Jerusalem artichoke	ac
All other vegetables	AL

MELONS

All melons	AL

SEEDS AND NUTS

All seeds and nuts	ac

SUGARS, FATS, AND OILS

Honey	AL
Olive oil	AL
Soy oil	AL
Sunflower oil	ac
Sesame oil	ac
Corn oil	AL
Avocado oil	AL
Brown sugar	ac
White sugar	ac
Milk sugar	ac
Maple syrup	ac
Cane syrup	ac
Malt syrup	ac
Blackstrap molasses	ac
Butter and margarine	ac
Cream	ac
All nut oils	ac

CARBOHYDRATES

Lima beans	AL
Parsnips	AL
Corn	AL
Potatoes, white	AL
Potatoes, sweet	AL
Millet	AL
Buckwheat	AL
Dried split Peas	ac
Beans of any kind	ac
Bread	ac
Bread made from sprouts	AL
Rice, white	ac

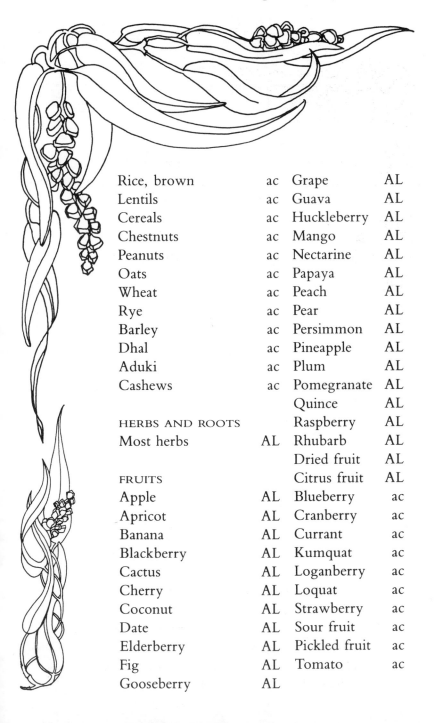

Rice, brown	ac	Grape	AL
Lentils	ac	Guava	AL
Cereals	ac	Huckleberry	AL
Chestnuts	ac	Mango	AL
Peanuts	ac	Nectarine	AL
Oats	ac	Papaya	AL
Wheat	ac	Peach	AL
Rye	ac	Pear	AL
Barley	ac	Persimmon	AL
Dhal	ac	Pineapple	AL
Aduki	ac	Plum	AL
Cashews	ac	Pomegranate	AL
		Quince	AL
		Raspberry	AL
HERBS AND ROOTS		Rhubarb	AL
Most herbs	AL	Dried fruit	AL
		Citrus fruit	AL
FRUITS		Blueberry	ac
Apple	AL	Cranberry	ac
Apricot	AL	Currant	ac
Banana	AL	Kumquat	ac
Blackberry	AL	Loganberry	ac
Cactus	AL	Loquat	ac
Cherry	AL	Strawberry	ac
Coconut	AL	Sour fruit	ac
Date	AL	Pickled fruit	ac
Elderberry	AL	Tomato	ac
Fig	AL		
Gooseberry	AL		

HERBAL LOW-CAL RECIPES

The following recipes from my *Herbal Guide to Inner Health* will give you a sampling of the herbal low-cal delights you can create in your own kitchen. Be creative, and experiment!

NASTURTIUM SALAD

1	large handful young Nasturtium leaves
1	large handful Lettuce leaves
	Some Watercress
	Some Sprouts
3 or 4	Spring Onions, sliced diagonally

Wash the salad greens, roll in a clean towel, and refrigerate for a few hours. Then take the greens and tear them into bite-size pieces into a bowl. Add the Watercress, Sprouts, and Spring Onions.

Dressing
Salad oil (Olive and Safflower)
Lemon juice
Honey
Salt
Pepper
Marigold petals
Some Nasturtium flowers

Shake over the salad some oil (to taste, probably about ¼ cup), and toss lightly. Mix the rest of the dressing ingredients (about ⅛ cup), shake over the salad, and again toss lightly. Decorate with the Nasturtium flowers. Yum, yum. It has a delicious, fresh, slightly hot flavor. This salad is very good when served as an accompaniment to a bland main course, such as Mushrooms on toast. The salad is excellent as a cleanser for the liver. (SERVES 4.)

FRESH MINT SALAD

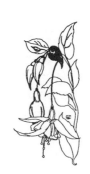

Watercress
Romaine Lettuce
Spring Onions
Nasturtium leaves and flowers
Spearmint
Chickweed

Take any assortment and quantity of the greens, wash and drain them, wrap in a clean terrycloth towel, and refrigerate. When ready to serve, tear the greens into bite-size pieces and fill a salad bowl with your assortment.

For a Simple Dressing, sprinkle Safflower oil over the greens. This particular salad requires a lighter-tasting oil than Olive oil. You could also try Soybean oil. Toss the salad. Just before serving, add salt and Pepper and toss lightly again. Add a tablespoon or two of Tarragon-flavored vinegar or Lemon juice and toss again.

VEGETABLE SALAD SUPREME

It is really a mistake to give a particular set of ingredients for a vegetable salad because the makings for one of these truly depends on the contents of your refrigerator or your garden. I would hate it if you felt you had to go shopping every time you wanted to make one of my recipes. So please just poke around your house or garden for the herbs, investigate your refrigerator for vegetables, and check out the empty lot next door or search the countryside for some fresh greens. Wash what you've collected, drain it, dry it, tear or cut it into pieces, and put it together in a bowl. Then top with a drizzle of good oil and a squeeze of Lemon juice, toss with a handful of minced herbs, serve it on lovely salad plates, and eat! One of my recent vegetable salads consisted of diagonally sliced Zucchini, finely sliced red Cabbage, diagonally sliced Cucumber, and diagonally sliced Celery all arranged on a plate. Then I added some sliced Tomato, sprinkled on some Soybean sprouts, and put on some Avocado slices. I composed the dressing as I went along: a drizzle of Safflower oil, a grand sprinkling of dried Chervil and other herbs, and then squeezed half a Lemon over all, and added a touch of Tarragon-flavored white wine vinegar. I looked at the salad and liked it, but then decided to add some Alfalfa sprouts and some flowers (Nasturtiums and Violets) for color. It was delicious.

GARLIC SOUP

6–24	Garlic cloves (about 1–4 bulbs)
2	T or more good quality Olive oil
1	qt rich chicken or vegetable broth or stock
3	egg yolks
	Chopped Parsley, yogurt, ground Almonds, optional

Crush the Garlic cloves with the flat of a knife and slip off skins. Sauté the Garlic slowly in oil in a cast-iron skillet until translucent. Add the broth or stock (that means liquid only, no solids or blended foods), and simmer gently about 20 minutes until the Garlic is mushy. Press the Garlic-broth blend through a ricer or sieve, or squeeze through coarse cheesecloth into a bowl. Beat the egg yolks until thick with a wire whisk in a 2-quart enamel or stainless-steel pot. Then beat in slowly, a teaspoon at a time, some of the warm Garlic broth. Beat in about 3 tablespoons altogether. (What we are trying to do here is warm th egg yolks without cooking them.) Combine the 2 mixtures slowly, heat to boiling, and serve in wide soup plates.

This soup can be a delicious first course of a meal—just add dollops of chopped Parsley, yogurt, and ground Almonds to the soup when it is served.

The soup is mainly seasoned by the broth. If you wish, add any of the following depending on the results you wish to obtain: salt, Pepper, Cayenne, Oregano, or Parsley.

MY FIFTH VEGETABLE SOUP

I have a friend who quite casually suggested that I try vegetarianism. He made the point that for someone who lectured as much as I did about the virtues of the diet, I should at least try it or stop talking about it. So I did, but it was somewhat difficult. I am the product of a French mother and had never before tried to make soup without at least a delicious marrow bone. The first soups I tried were okay, but this one was delicious, although the ingredients may seem a little bit odd.

1	red Onion, sliced
4	or more Greek cloves, whole and peeled
	Celery tops, chopped
1	Sweet Potato, halved and sliced
2	Carrots, sliced
	Some sliced Cabbage
1	green hot Chile Pepper, sliced
	Olive oil
1	bottle (3–4 cups) hearty burgundy
1–2	qt water
1	Tomato, quartered
	Small handful Calendula petals
1	t Korean Mint, crushed
½	t crushed Coriander seeds
1	piece (1–2 inches) Cinnamon stick
1	T all-purpose herb blend

Sauté all the vegetables together in some Olive oil until the potato is slightly browned. Add the hearty burgundy, water, Tomato, Calendula, and spices. Simmer together for an hour. Let age and meld for a few hours or overnight before reheating and serving. You may want to add some Dulse, Kelp, or salt before serving. This soup is delicious with some sourdough French bread and a huge, delicious vegetable salad. (SERVES 4–8.)

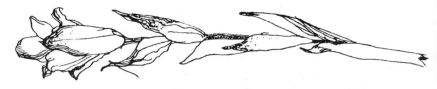

CHINESE-STYLE STEAMED FISH

4–5	lb red snapper or other firm, white-fleshed fish
	Azuki beans, cooked and salted
1/8	cup Chinese rice wine
1	Onion, sliced
1/8	cup toasted Sesame oil
1/4	cup good quality Soy sauce
1	piece fresh Ginger
2	Garlic cloves, crushed
	Szechuan Peppercorns, crushed
1	red Chile, optional
4	Spring Onions with tops, sliced diagonally
	Fresh Cilantro (Coriander tops, Chinese Parsley)

Clean the fish, leaving the head on. Wash the fish thoroughly inside and out and dry it. Rub the inside of the fish with salted Azuki beans. Mix the wine, Onion, Sesame oil, Soy sauce, Ginger, Garlic, Szechuan Peppercorns, and Chile. Pour this mixture over the fish and soak it for several hours.

Use a pan with a rack to hold the fish at least 1 inch off the bottom of the pan. Put the fish in the pan, belly side down with the sides opened out. Pour over it the soaking mixture. Cover the pan and steam it over medium heat for about 20–40 minutes until almost done. Meanwhile diagonally slice the Spring Onions and tear up some fresh Cilantro. Put half of this mixture over the fish and steam for 15 more minutes, or until done. To test, insert a fork: The flesh will flake when done. Place the fish on an attractive serving platter with the rest of the Onion and Cilantro decoratively covering the top. Add more Soy sauce and crushed Garlic if you wish. (SERVES 8.)

STEAK TARTARE

1	lb ground steak
1	handful minced Parsley
1/2	Lemon, juiced
2–4	Garlic cloves, pressed
1	egg yolk, beaten frothy
1/4	cup minced Onion (or more)
1	t Dijon-type Mustard, hot
1	T drained Capers or pickled Nasturtium seedpods
1	T anchovies, freshly chopped
	Seasonings (all or some, to your taste):
1	T Olive oil
1	t Worcestershire sauce or Outerbridge's Sherry-Pepper sauce
	Salt
	Freshly ground Pepper
	Dash of hot sauce (like Tabasco)

Get the very best quality steak (use lean meat and cuts known as eye round, top sirloin, or top round) and have it ground to order. Mix everything. Shape this into a nice round mound, refrigerate until chilled, and serve as an hors d'oeuvre with a robust red wine and crackers. A good food if you are protein-deficient and carnivorous by nature.

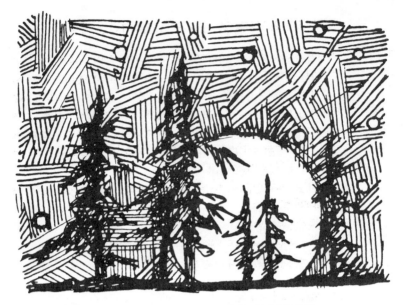

YOGURT-GARLIC SAUCE

1–4	Garlic cloves
	Salt or powdered Kelp
1/2	cup Yogurt
	Goodly pinch of herb, rubbed between the palms (herb depends on what the sauce is for)
	Some Suggested Combinations:
	Mint with lamb
	Dill or Fennel with fish
	Basil with Tomatoes or over cottage cheese
	Chives or Parsley with eggs
	Sage, Lemon, or Tarragon for chicken

Finely chop the Garlic and pound it with a pestle in a mortar. Add the salt and pound to a paste, while slowly adding the yogurt. When it is really smooth, taste the mix and add more salt if necessary. Stir in the herb.

Besides the uses mentioned above, this yogurt-Garlic sauce is excellent to eat by itself for disordered digestion, and it can be applied to insect bites or some skin irritations. (MAKES ⅔ CUP.)

SHIRLEY'S SALSA MEXICANA

This delicious sauce always accompanies meals in Mexico. It is served over breakfast eggs, seafood, steaks, and other meals. Tacos are improvised with tortillas, fresh or fried, bits of chicken, cheese, or any leftover meat and *Salsa Mexicana*. It is thought to cleanse the digestive system, ridding the intestines of parasites and amoebas—those troublesome ailments referred to as "Montezuma's Revenge."

    2   cups chopped fresh Tomatoes (skinned, if you prefer)
    3/4 cup chopped Onion
    2   T chopped hot green Chile Peppers
    1   T chopped Cilantro
    1   t salt
         Juice of 2 Limes

Combine all ingredients and refrigerate before serving to allow the flavors to blend. (Courtesy of Shirley Boccaccio.)

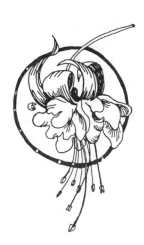

7

...

Today's Indoor Herb Garden

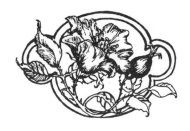

During the last part of the sixties I lived in a third-floor walk-up apartment near the famous, or infamous (depending on how you perceive it), Haight-Ashbury district of San Francisco. It was the kind of apartment called a railroad flat because all the rooms were in a line, one after the other. As you entered the front door you would have seen an infinitesimally small living room to the left where I first began to teach classes in herbology. Straight across from the front door was an even smaller kitchen, once photographed by the *Village Voice,* that had a short shelf with some of my herbal products and experiments. Down the hall was the bathroom, an enlarged part of the hall euphemistically called the office, where I wrote *Herbs and Things,* and then the bedroom/sewing room/magic room/artist's loft. This last room was large and went through various transformations through the years, once even becoming a kennel for six Great Dane puppies that I raised and nursed by hand from their birth. Through the door of this sunny room was a pathetically small back porch about 5 feet by 5 feet where I raised all my herbs in tiers and layers that had to be manually raised and lowered so that they would all reach the sun at least a part of every day. This pitiful bunch of potted plants became the beginnings of the burgeoning herb garden I have today.

CARE

Herbs are notoriously difficult to raise in pots. When they are actually rooted in the ground, they seem to require no more than benign neglect. When incarcerated in a clay pot, however, moisture, plenty of sunlight, tender care, good nutrition, plenty of attention, and time are all absolutely necessary. Although all of these things were hard to come by in my youth, my plants prospered and flourished. When I was finally able to put them into the ground in 1971, they grew tall in a very short time.

When growing herbs in pots you must remember two main things: Water before the soil dries out or before the leaves yellow and fall off, and use soil that is a touch on the alkaline side and that has excellent drainage. Herbs grown indoors are generally grown for their scent and the excellence of their taste, both of which are a result of the quality and quantity of the volatile oils in their leaves. With artificially fertilized moist soil you may get a plant that looks hearty and green, but it will leave much to be desired in the taste and scent category. So neglect those indoor herb plants a little, but not a lot. I both fertilize and water my plants simultaneously with herb water. This stuff is easy to make and is also an excellent conditioner for the more traditional house plants.

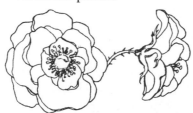

J.R.'S FAMOUS HERBAL WATER
(TO WATER AND FERTILIZE)

5	gal water (an old glass or plastic water bottle will do)
2	lb Comfrey leaf, chopped, either dried or fresh, some root also okay
2	lb Dandelion leaf, chopped, fresh or dried (pick it out of the garden)—this plant alkalinizes
1/2	lb Nettle leaf, chopped, fresh or dried

Add the herbs to the water and let infuse at least 3 days before using to water the plants. Use only half the water and then refill the container with fresh water from the tap or with rainwater that you have collected. You may continue to add water to this container, as it is used up until the herbs can no longer color the water. Finally you will have a mass of decaying matter left in the bottom of the container, which will make an excellent fertilizer for any plant you have growing indoors or out. Just put a layer on the surface of the soil and dig it in a bit.

Indoor herb plants need plenty of light and warmth. Grow them in a window that has southern exposure. I grew Tuberose indoors and never failed to get manificent blossoms that scented the room wonderfully when the sun was able to penetrate San Francisco's notorious fog. But the quantity of sunlight was not enough to keep the stems strong. The poor Tuberose had to be carefully staked and tied at intervals during the growing season to hold them up long enough to produce flowers.

You can also grow herbs outdoors on a scrawny back porch and bring them inside regularly to brighten your day. They can be shifted about, from outside to inside, from room to room as the patterns and strength of the sunlight change from one season to the next. Light of the natural or artificial sort can keep the fragrant herbs growing all year.

Herbs do not like wet roots, except for herbs like Calamus and Ginger rhizomes. It's best to keep a layer of clean pebbles in the bottom of your drainage saucer to keep the roots from getting soggy, which will cause rot. While we are talking about Calamus we should mention that the best way to grow any plant is to reproduce its natural habitat as closely as possible. Check in a plant identification book for your plant's normal habitat and manner of growth and then mimic this within the limits of your own environment. The Calamus, for instance, needs to grow in nice boggy swamplike conditions. I keep mine in the bathroom, which has a southern exposure with a few hours of sunlight a day and indirect light the rest of the time. I use a clay pot without drainage holes and keep an inch of water covering the rhizome at all times. It has grown 4 feet tall. I started Ginger from a piece purchased in the grocery store, potted it in rich potting soil, watered it constantly during the spring and summer, and after it had flowered, I let it dry out and stored it in the dark until the following year.

Herb plants should be grown only in clay pots, even though clay pots are porous and can discolor tabletops and windowsills with water rings. So hide the plain clay pot in attractive containers such as baskets or exotic tins like those sold containing Italian Olive oil or cookies. Nonporous china or glass containers are also nice.

Potting soil can be purchased at any nursery or made to order. Just follow directions from some good gardening manual. I personally use only two such books, *How to Grow Herbs,* a Sunset Book from Lane Books in Menlo Park, California, and a wonderful Ortho book, *The World of Herbs and Spices* (available in nurseries or by writing to Ortho Books, 575 Market Street, San Francisco, CA 94105). I like the Ortho Book best because of the beautiful photographs, all of which are in color. You can make your own all-purpose potting soil by mixing equal parts of store-bought potting soil, peat moss, herb mixture (rotted and chopped Comfrey, Nettle, Dandelion, and Kelp), and vermiculite (for drainage).

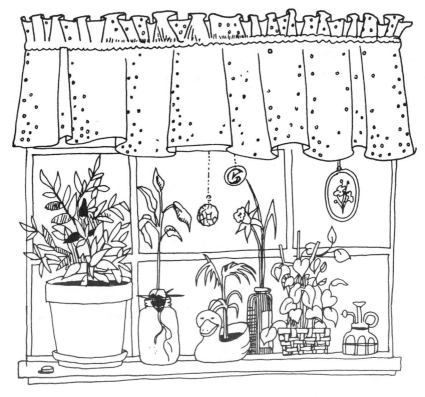

Vegetables can also be grown indoors by using fluorescent-style tubing of full-spectrum light to supplement natural sunlight. Install a 4-foot reflector-type fixture that will hold standard fluorescent tubes in a window or under a cabinet. Use 40-watt tubes of full-spectrum light. Use any sort of container, making sure there are drainage holes and something to catch the overflow. The container should be at least 10–15 inches deep so that vegetable roots can grow long and strong. Plant the seeds and simply follow the directions on the seed package. Fertilize the plants with J.R.'s Famous Herbal Water once a week.

Insects on house plants, potted vegetables, or herb plants can be treated with a homemade insecticide.

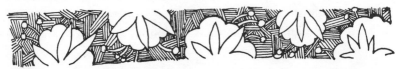

SMELLY ONION INSECTICIDE
FOR WHITE FLY AND APHIDS

1   gal bottle
2   chopped Onions
2   chopped Garlic bulbs (not cloves)
    Enough water to cover

Leave this to ferment for several weeks. When good and smelly, strain through cheesecloth into a sprinkling-type bottle with large holes or into a container used to dispense talcum powder. Sprinkle plants every 3–4 days until the problem is controlled.

OIL-BASED SPRAY FOR SCALE

2   cups Pyrethrum flowers, fresh-picked, sun-dried, and then ground to powder
    Enough Sesame oil to just cover the powdered flowers

Leave to ferment in a hot place for 2 weeks, then strain carefully through cheesecloth. Paint the oil on plants troubled with scale or sprinkle on with some sort of sprinkling can. Pyrethrum is a contact insecticide available in most garden stores. It can be used freely on plants since it is only harmful to invertebrate creatures. You can use the powdered flowers as a dust or make a water-based spray or use as above as an oil-based spray. The Sesame oil works with the Pyrethrum to increase its effectiveness.

House plants have to be grown according to their own needs. Many books and charts giving specific growing needs for each type of house plant are available. In my own home I grow a few cacti and other special plants I have nurtured for years. Although I prefer to see plants in their natural habitat, it's comforting and pleasant to always be surrounded by greenery. I

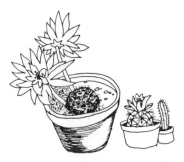

keep my indoor plants healthy by spraying occasionally with the Pyrethrum or Onion spray. I'm attentive to their light and moisture needs and mulch them regularly.

I have a mixture of Fennel seed and Comfrey root that my family uses as a first-aid remedy (see p. 178). Since this is made every third day I have a constant supply of wet infused Fennel seeds and Comfrey root. This herbal sticky stuff has been added to the soil of a San Pedro cactus growing near my kitchen. The growth of this succulent over the last three years has been phenomenal. Whenever I make herbal concoctions or herbal baths, do you think I throw out the roots and seeds after the water has extracted their goodness? Absolutely not. This solid matter is used on all my house plants as a natural source of nourishment, an herbal food, if you will, to provide minerals and vitamins to keep the plants healthy.

In caring for indoor house plants, whether herbs, vegetables, or the more traditional house plant, you should always pay close attention to:

Moisture needs
Direction and amount of light
pH and quality of the soil
Type of soil, its density, whether sand or clay (i.e., its ability to
    drain or retain fluid)

And remember the general rule of thumb that whenever possible you should try to reproduce the conditions under which the plant grows in its natural environment.

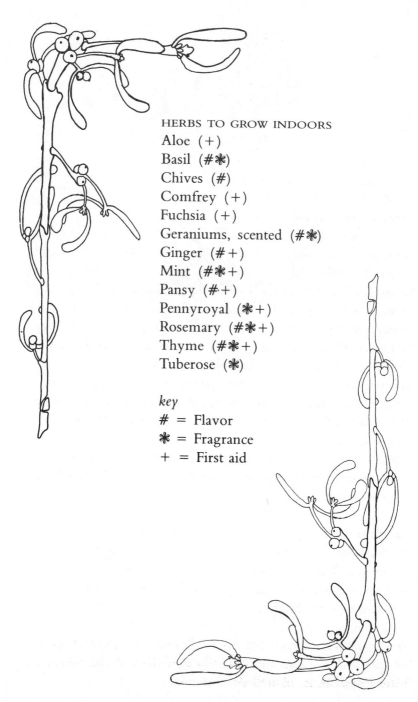

HERBS TO GROW INDOORS
Aloe (+)
Basil (#✳)
Chives (#)
Comfrey (+)
Fuchsia (+)
Geraniums, scented (#✳)
Ginger (#+)
Mint (#✳+)
Pansy (#+)
Pennyroyal (✳+)
Rosemary (#✳+)
Thyme (#✳+)
Tuberose (✳)

key
= Flavor
✳ = Fragrance
+ = First aid

8

· · ·

The Herbal Pet

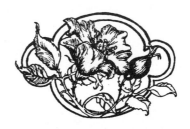

Taking care of your pets should be very much like taking care of your children. Their health is totally dependent on the master's whim and knowledge. Animals, however, do not need continual care as they will actually prosper with a certain amount of benign neglect. Give them an excellent diet with inspired nutrition, which should free them from both internal and external parasites and keep them in good health, add a generous quantity of exercise and a healthy dose of love and you will have an animal without neuroses or physical problems.

Animal care has more to do with proper diet than anything else. An animal that is allowed free access to the outside will generally get enough exercise to stay in good health, but it is your responsibility to see that the diet is superior. Still, illness will occur and has to be treated and the intelligent owner with a little foresight and knowledge can save many trips to the veterinary not to mention saving money.

DIET

What one eats is of great importance. Diet can be the difference between vibrant active health and weakness. Wild animals eating their natural diet suffer very little from disease. Feed your pets commercial food alone and disease is probably inevitable. Feed them a commercial diet plus vitamin and mineral supplements and disease is less likely, but feed them a homemade food made from scratch from wholesome, nutritious, unsprayed ingredients and your pets will have the resistance and stamina to fight off any disease that may come along.

HOMEMADE DIET

	Cats	Dogs
Meat (especially organ meats like heart, kidney, or liver)—raw, chopped or slightly sautéed	50%	30%
Muscle meats, fish and eggs—raw or slightly cooked	10%	10%
Grains, especially sprouted grains such as Wheat, Oats, Millet, Rice, or Barley	25%	40%
Food supplements such as milk powder, Wheat germ and brewer's yeast flakes	5%	5%
Vegetables, especially Carrots, Beets, dark green or dark yellow vegetables—grated, raw or chopped and slightly cooked	10%	15%
Fruit (feed only as a treat)		
Herbal supplements		
Vitamin and mineral supplements		

Mix the ingredients, depending on what grains and vegetables you have available. Make thick patties like hamburger patties, separate them with wax paper and freeze what you don't need immediately.

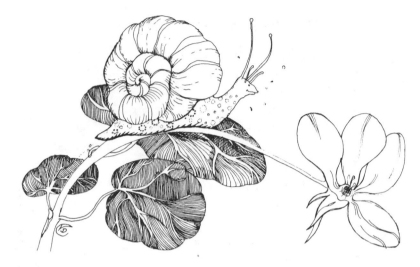

Occasionally, feed your cats and dogs muscle meat; but since there is substantially more nutrition in organ meats these are to be preferred. Fruits should be fed only as a treat. My Abyssinian cats adore Cantaloupe, so they get this fruit when it is in season and Corn on the cob when it is available. But these foods are not given on a regular basis. My Great Dane adored Avocadoes and he got this delectable fruit several times a month. The amount that you feed depends on the size of the animal and how much exercise it gets. The best way to determine how much to feed your pet is to feed it all that it can eat twice a day remembering to remove leftovers after 30 minutes.

Always leave plenty of water available. Supplements should be fed at every meal—1–3 teaspoons per day is adequate for most cats and 1 tablespoon to 1 cup (depending on the animal's size) will take care of a dog.

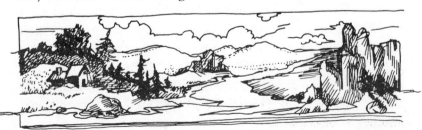

HERBAL SUPPLEMENTS

1	oz Alfalfa
1/4	oz Burdock root or seed
1/2	oz Camomile
1/4	oz Catnip
	dash Cayenne
1	oz Comfrey
1	oz Dandelion
1/4	oz Fennel seeds
1/4	oz Garlic
1/2	Horsetail
1	oz Marshmallow root
1	oz Mullen leaf
1	oz Nettle
1/2	oz Oatstraw
1	oz Parsley
1/2	Red Clover
1/2	oz Rose hips
1/2	oz Rosemary
1/2	oz Slippery Elm
1/2	oz Thyme

Directions: Start only with dried, cut up, chopped, or powdered herbs. Mix them all together. Put the entire lot through a blender or chopper to reduce to a coarse powder. Store in a dark jar in the refrigerator or in a cool place. Use the herbal supplement mixed in the food or sprinkled on the top of the food. For a nursing or pregnant mother add to the above mixture ½ ounce each of Milk Thistle, Raspberry leaf, Chickweed, and another ½ ounce of Comfrey.

AILMENTS

Feed your pet pure, wholesome food and you can skip the rest of this chapter. But if it just happens to get sick here are some useful formulas that will help you treat simple symptoms and illnesses.

How do you tell if your pet is sick? Check for these signs: breath; pulse; clarity of the eye; smell of the body, nose, ears, hindquarters; temperature of the internal body as well as the temperature of the skin and limbs; integrity of the skin and quality of the hair or fur; posture or stance; and presence or absence of pain in any part of the body.

If any of these signs seem abnormal there is a possibility that the pet is sick. Once my Great Dane came to me and kept nudging me with his massive head. I looked at him and checked him thoroughly and could find nothing wrong. I finally came to his mouth to check his breath to see whether or not it was offensive and upon opening his mouth the problem was readily apparent. The dog had gotten into a neighbor's garbage and had gotten a dog food can lid wedged in his mouth between his upper teeth. I removed the lid and medicated the cuts on the gum and he was fine. But never ignore an animal that is bothering you, as it just might have something physically wrong.

PARASITES

Internal parasites can be effectively removed with the following formulation.

1. Fast the animal for 24 hours and bury all feces. Give an enema if possible.
2. Feed large quantities of Garlic every hour. Either chop it up and put into small quantities of meat or take whole cloves and put them down the animal's throat.

3. Feed the animal a worming mixture made from equal quantities of finely chopped or powdered Thyme, Garlic, and Wormwood. Give capsules of this mixture—1 for every 10 pounds plus a laxative preceding the capsule (like milk of magnesia), an enema after the bowel movement, and a pure wholesome diet emphasizing wholesome raw foods.

External parasites can be dealt with, with a diet that has plenty of B vitamins, extra supplements of brewer's yeast, clean bedding that has been laundered with Pennyroyal herb, and herbal sleep pillows to act as a deterrent to the fleas.

CAT AND DOG SLEEP PILLOWS
(Flea Repellent)

Cat

2	oz Pennyroyal
1	oz Catnip
1	oz Camomile

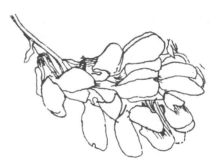

Dog

2	oz Pennyroyal
1	oz Thyme
1	oz Wormwood

Use whole or cut herbs and stuff the mixture into a large pillow (2 feet by 2 feet for a cat and 3 feet by 3 feet or larger for a dog) made of a tough cloth such as denim.

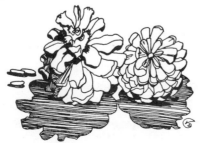

FLEA POWDER
(For Cats and Dogs)

2   oz Pennyroyal
1   oz Wormwood
     large dash Cayenne
1   oz Rosemary

Use these herbs in powdered form. Mix them. Store in a container. Use whenever necessary as you would any type of body powder.

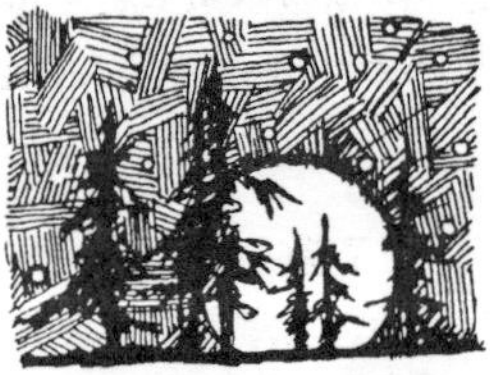

SORES AND ABSCESSES

Abrasions, sores, or abscesses are common in pets that are allowed freedom to run. An abscess, which Cats are especially susceptible to, is a collection of pus under the skin surrounded by inflamed tissue, usually caused by a scratch or bite that has become infected. All of these surface and deeper irritations can be treated at home with a few simple remedies.

CLEANSING TONIC FOR ALL ILLNESS

1   T Burdock
1   T Cayenne
2   T Goldenseal
1   T Garlic
1   T Chaparral

Start with dried herbs that are finely powdered. Mix these herbs thoroughly. Stuff the powder into gelatin capsules (0—single-aught size) and feed 1 capsule for every 10 pounds every 3 hours. Feed your pet no more than 5 doses in a day.

EXTERNAL FOMENTATION OR WASH

Mix equal quantities of Camomile, Comfrey root, Red Clover, and Thyme. They can be fresh or dried, whole or cut. Make a strong infusion and use as a fomentation. Dip a muslin or woolen cloth in the strong infusion and apply to the sore or irritated areas. Keep the herbal liquid hot throughout the course of treatment.

The heat of a fomentation will help to bring the infection to the surface. The scab can then be removed from the abscess so that it can drain. When the wound has opened sprinkle Goldenseal powder on it, which will act as an antibacterial.

EXTERNAL OR INTERNAL ANTIBACTERIAL POWDER
(Mange or Hair Loss)

Mix equal quantities of dried powdered Garlic and Goldenseal. Keep this in your first-aid kit and apply freely to any sore or abraded area where bacteria might become a problem.

Any simple scratch, burn, slight abrasion, irritated pad, or bitten ear can be simply treated. Wash the area carefully with soap and water and apply Comfrey gel.

COMFREY GEL

Either purchase comfrey gel in a container or make it by simmering freshly chopped Comfrey root in an equal quantity of water for about 20 minutes. Let the mixture cool and strain through a coarse screen. The gel can be used immediately or it can be rolled into small balls and frozen for future use.

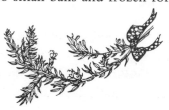

SPRAINS AND RHEUMATISM

Many pets suffer from the same type of rheumatic pains that humans do and the treatment is similar. Rosemary, Comfrey leaf and root, Devil's claw, and Rooibos can be added to the diet as a supplementary food and tincture of Arnica as an external application. Tincture of Arnica can be purchased at any pharmacy. Homeopathic grains of Arnica is also a simple, useful first-aid treatment for a sprain or rheumatic tightness.

TINCTURE OF ARNICA

8   oz Arnica herb
8   oz alcohol (rubbing alcohol is good, as are gin or vodka)

Soak 4 ounces of the Arnica in the alcohol, macerating for about 10 days. Daily mash and stir the herb into the alcohol. At the end of the 10 days carefully strain the mixture through coarse muslin, squeezing the herb until it is almost dry. Discard the herb and to the alcohol add another 4 ounces of Arnica and repeat the process. At the end of the 20 days you will have about 7 ounces of Arnica tincture. Bottle it in a dark glass jar or container, label it carefully, and use as a friction rub or application to sprains, strains, and bruises.

EYES AND EARS

Animals often get irritants into their eyes and ears. These can generally be managed with a simple wash to cleanse the eye or ear and a soothing application of an emolient herb to heal.

EYEWASH

Use 1 tablespoon of Comfrey root and 1 tablespoon of Fennel seed in cut or crushed form. They can be dried or fresh. Mix the herbs, put into a small pot, and add 4 ounces of water. Bring to a boil, remove from the heat and let the mixture steep until cool. Strain through a fine strainer or silk, bottle in glass, and refrigerate.

This wash can beused by anyone in the household to wash and heal the eyes. Actually it is a superior first-aid wash for any irritations, cuts, scratches, burns, or bites.

The ears can be washed out with the eyewash and lubricated with Mullein oil. Mullein oil is now being made by many companies and is available in health food stores. It can also be made at home very simply with Mullein flowers and Olive oil. This oil has superior healing and soothing qualities for earache or ear mites and as an application when foxtails have been removed. Another healing application for the ear is a Garlic oil perle squeezed directly into the ear canal.

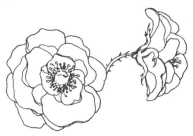

MULLEIN OIL

4   oz dried or fresh Mullein flowers
       enough Olive oil to just cover the flowers

Cover the flowers with the Olive oil and make sure that the flowers do not float above the oil. Stir the mixture daily for 10 days and then strain carefully through silk cloth.

CLEANLINESS

A clean animal will generally be a healthy animal. Brush cats and dogs daily to remove loose hairs, sprinkle flea powder on them once a week to deter fleas, and once a month give a bath using a natural Olive oil castile soap or Rosemary Soap.

ROSEMARY SOAP

1   grated bar of castile soap
3   oz infusion of Rosemary herb

Melt the soap in the top of a double boiler and add the infusion at any time. When the soap is melted, stir everything until incorporated. Pour the soap into a wide-mouth container and let it set.

This is a good soap to use to deter parasites and to keep the skin clean.

ROSEMARY OIL SOAP SPOT REMOVER

1   grated bar of castile soap
1   oz Rosemary oil
1   oz alcohol

Melt the soap, add the oil and the alcohol, and mix. Pour into a wide-mouth container and let the mixture set. Use the soap as a spot remover on natural fabrics or rugs to remove urine or feces stains. The scent will also deter the animal from using that area again as a place to dump.

Digestive disturbances may be noticeable because the feces or the urine become particularly bad smelling. In cases like this, simplify the diet and add more vitamin and food supplements, such as Catnip and vitamin C, to the food.

FOR OFFENSIVE FECES

Add 1 tablespoon of Uva Ursi to every 3 cups of drinking water. Put the herb loose in the water or wrap it in a bit of muslin. This will act to deodorize the feces and urine by cleansing the digestive and excretory tract.

For any other problem of unknown origin it will not hurt to add the Cleansing Tonic formula that was mentioned earlier.

EXERCISE

Animals that are kept indoors do not exercise enough. They must be taken out, especially in the morning or the evening, and walked or run. Animals must exercise in all sorts of weather to really maintain vital health. Cats can generally be allowed to run loose in the backyard where they will climb trees, fight bushes, and joyously leap about. A dog needs to be taken out into the world, the park or the countryside, and really let free to jump and run. It is only through really vigorous exercise that the lungs can fill with oxygen, which is cleansing and invigorating to the respiratory system. All of the organs benefit from vigorous exercise.

HERBS MOST OFTEN USED IN ANIMAL CARE

Alfalfa (*Medicago sativa* L.)—dried, ground seeds; dried powdered, or cut herb

Burdock (*Arctium lappa* L.)—dried, ground seeds for the skin; dried, powdered, or cut root

Camomile (*Anthemis nobilis* L.)—dried or fresh, whole flowers

Catnip (*Nepeta cataria* L.)—fresh or dried, chopped or powdered herb

Cayenne (*Capsicum species* L.)—dried and powdered fruit without the seeds

Chaparral or Creosote Bush (*Larrea divaricata* Car.)—dried and cut herb

Chickweed (*Stellaria media* [L.] Cyr.)—dried or fresh, whole or cut herb

Comfrey (*Symphytum officinale* L.)—dried or fresh, cut or powdered herb, root, or both

Dandelion (*Taraxacum officinale* Wiggers)—dried or fresh, cut or powdered herb or root

Fennel (*Foeniculum vulgare* Mill.)—dried, whole, or powdered seeds

Garlic (*Allium sativum* L.)—dried, whole, powdered, crushed, or cut herb and cloves

Goldenseal (*Hydrastis canadensis* L.)—dried, powdered root

Horsetail (*Equisetum arvense*)—dried, powdered, or cut herb

Marshmallow (*Althaea officinalis* L.)—fresh or dried, powdered or cut herb and root

Milk Thistle (*Carduus marianus* or *Silybum marianum*)—fresh or dried, powdered or cut herb

Mullein (*Verbascum thapsus* L.)—fresh or dried, powdered or cut herb; whole or powdered flowers

Nettle (*Urtica dioica* L.)—dried, powdered, or cut herb

Oatstraw (*Avena sativa* L.)—dried, powdered, or cut Oat grass; dried, powdered, or cut herb

Parsley (*Petroselinum species*)—dried or fresh, powdered or cut, herb or root

Pennyroyal (*Mentha pulegium* L.)—dried, powdered, or cut herb

Raspberry (*Rubus idaeus* L.)—dried, powdered, or cut bark or herb

Red Clover (*Trifolium pratense* L.)—dried, powdered, or cut herb; whole flowers

Rose (*Rosa species* L.)—dried or fresh, powdered, cut, or whole hips

Rosemary (*Rosmarinus officinalis* L.)—dried or fresh, powdered or cut herb

Slippery Elm or Flaxseed (*Ulmus fulva* Michx. or *Linum usitatissimum*)—dried, powdered bark of Elm; dried, whole, or powdered seeds

Thyme (*Thymus vulgaris* L.)—dried or fresh, powdered or cut herb

Uva Ursi (*Arctostaphylos Uva-ursi* L.)—dried, powdered, or cut herb

Wormwood (*Artemisia absinthium* L.)—dried, powdered, or cut herb

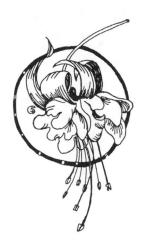

9
...
Sports Herbology

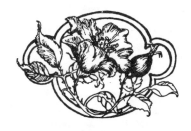

During the summer as well as other times, a variety of injuries can occur from sports activites. The most persistent problem facing athletes is common stiffness. During and after almost any exercise, lactic acid is released into the muscles in large quantities. Because it cannot be removed very efficiently or quickly, it causes pain. You know that feeling of tightness that you get the day after a bit of strenuous exercise? This is caused by the accumulation of lactic acid in the muscles. The only way to get rid of the lactic acid is to keep moving, keep exercising. As the lactic acid is released and metabolized over a couple of days the aching will also disappear. Continued exercise is as crucial to a weekend athlete as it is to a seasoned athlete. Exercise helps the body flush away the buildup of lactic acid.

There are herbs that help to flush away lactic acid and herbs that work on the cause, not the symptoms, of a particular pain. The addition of herbs and plants to the diet and their external application help restore the body's natural balance and relieve conditions that modern medicine often cannot affect.

But we must use these herbs diligently. One cup of tea will certainly not cure a broken ankle, but many cups of Comfrey root tea used externally and Comfrey leaf tea taken internally can speed the healing process immensely.

TRAINING

The best way to avoid aching muscles or a stretched or torn ligament is to get into condition. If you have been sitting around the office for 10 years and suddenly decide that you must begin a program of exercise that will make you the fit young thing you were at 16, for heaven's sake, *start slowly*. First stretch your body like a cat, each part individually to its fullest. If you are really out of shape start your return to vibrant health with walks or with a yoga class. It is madness to pick up a tennis racket after a long period away from the court and play 4 straight sets. You'll be in agony for 2 weeks.

Walk, jog, go to a "fat" farm for a week, take short hikes, but always warm up to your particular sport slowly. Don't play in the broiling sun or freezing sleet unless you are proficient in that particular sport. And don't forget to stretch out. The more flexible you are, the less prone you will be to tears and injuries. Work up to longer walks and faster jogging or longer swims. Eventually, after several months, you will have built up your body, slimmed your sagging rear and improved your game. Whatever the sport, certain muscles will be called into use more than others. The more you condition your entire body, the stronger you will be, all over. The more endurance you have, the more energy and the less chance of damaging injury.

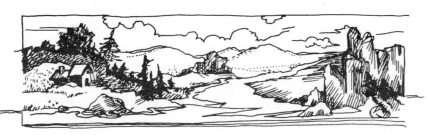

EMERGENCY CARE FOR
SPORTS-RELATED INJURIES

In sports medicine it is already assumed that your diet is optimum, that you are taking a variety of vitamin and mineral supplements to increase your endurance and reduce the stress on your body. If you want to perform to your utmost, take 1–3 tablespoons of brewer's yeast and especially bee pollen before a game or any physical activity. After a run or swim or any exercise take 1–3 tablespoons of Wheat germ oil in a glass of skim milk. These supplements are well known to build endurance and promote health.

If you have overexercised and your poor muscles are screaming in pain as a result of lactic acid buildup, drink a cup of Saffron (not Safflower) tea. Several cups before exercise and several cups for several days after will help keep you ache-free. Saffron has the ability to neutralize lactic acid by quickly moving it from the muscles to the liver where the body alchemically changes it to glycogen. Glycogen is then pumped out to the body and used for more energy. Saffron, although expensive, is so useful for this that you ought to think about purchasing it by the ounce rather than the gram. At the time of this writing good Saffron cost about $60 per ounce from a wholesaler, although you should be able to purchase the less expensive Saffron dust.

A substance that I have found particularly effective in relieving all sorts of aches and pains is DMSO (dimethylsulfoxide). It really has magical properties and can be mixed with *pure* essential oils to make the oils more penetrating. It can also be painted onto the aching spot for relief within 20 minutes. DMSO may be used along with the Saffron tea and herbal poultices to promote the healing of torn, sore, or aching muscles. (See page 29 for more information about DMSO.)

For relief of sore or bruised muscles, aching back or shoulders, bursitis, arthritis, aching joints, and other degenerative disorders, try this remedy.

ED SMITH'S CASTOR OIL PACK

3   layers of wool flannel
Castor oil
Pyrex pan
Plastic wrap or bag
Cotton towel
Hot pad

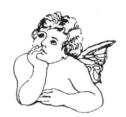

Soak flannel in enough Castor oil to thoroughly wet it. Put the soaked flannel in the pyrex pan into a 325-degree oven until thoroughly heated. Wring out the flannel to get rid of excess oil and wrap this around the sore or bruised area. Then wrap plastic around the flannel so that it won't leak. Wrap a towel or thick cloth around the plastic to keep in the heat and cover the whole thing with a hot pad set on medium. Do this for 1 hour about 3 times per week.

The soaked flannel can be kept and reused for quite some time. Eventually, the cloth gets hard from the oil and has to be discarded and new cloth soaked. For inflammation, a cold clay pack can be put on the skin first and then the hot Castor oil pack. For aching shoulders or back get a complete massage from an expert who can also judiciously apply moxa.

Herbal baths are also very effective in relieving the aches and pains of a tired, overexercised body. There are many herbs that can be used, such as Sage, Mugwort, Comfrey, Elder, Marshmallow root, Southernwood, Thyme, Lavender, Camomile, and especially Rosemary. Rosemary and Lavender are specifically for the muscles and joints and can always be used together. All of these herbs can also be used directly as a poultice or compress on injuries, or they can be mixed to be used in soaking baths. When you shower after any exercise and want to refresh yourself, wrap these herbs in muslin and scrub yourself with the bag as if it were a bar of soap. Don't rinse off the herbal waters that flow from the herb bag; let the water dry on your body for its soothing effect.

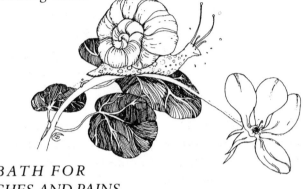

HERBAL BATH FOR
MUSCLE ACHES AND PAINS

Put equal parts of Sage, Mugwort, and Comfrey root into 1 quart of water in a covered nonmetal container. Use a large handful of the mixed herbs. Bring the mixture to a boil, then simmer the herbs gently for 10 minutes. Strain out the liquid and pour it into a tub of warm water; wrap the herbs in a piece of muslin or a cloth bag and use this bag to massage the body (it can also be applied as a compress to any sore spot after you take your bath).

When you take an herbal bath, especially for muscular ache, drink tea while bathing. This will relax you and help the herbs to work. It is also a good idea to use a cup of Epsom salts in the bath water to help bring toxins to the surface. So take an herbal/ Epsom salt bath, drink Peppermint or Comfrey tea (or a mixture of these herbs), soak for 20 minutes in the warming herbal waters, rub yourself with the bag of herbs, wrap yourself in a large towel, and read a book about proper conditioning for exercise.

Another bath mixture is Elder, Rosemary, and Thyme or Sassafras, each of which (or a combination) is excellent to help relax sore, tired, or strained muscles. The American Indians used Sassafras specifically for external relief of muscular fatigue, aches, and pains.

MUSCLE MIXTURE FOR BATH OR MASSAGE OIL

Formula 1:   Comfrey root, Agrimony, Sage, Mugwort, Burdock root, and Sassafras

Formula 2:   Comfrey root, Agrimony, Sage, Mugwort, Pennyroyal, and Wintergreen or Birch bark

Both of these formulas are very effective either used as an herbal mixture for the bath or infused in a good-quality oil and used as a massage oil. (Both formulas are available from the Herbal BodyWorks, 219 Carl Street, San Francisco, CA 94117.)

For the massage oil, simmer 2 ounces of the mixed herbs in a quart of oil for 20 minutes. Use a double boiler if possible. If you simmer them directly over the heat, watch the pot closely so that the herbs won't burn in the hot oil. After 20 minutes, turn off the heat and let the herbs steep in the oil until cool. Then turn on the heat again, bring the oil to a light boil, and simmer again, very gently, for another 20 minutes. Turn off the heat and cool again until it is possible to strain. Place some cheesecloth or muslin in a strainer and pour the oil through the cloth into another container. The oil will be a nice green color. Let it stand for a few days while it settles. The plant dyes and debris will settle out. Decant the clear green oil into a quart-size bottle. Scent formula number 1 with oil of Sassafras and number 2 with essential oil of Wintergreen. The first oil is a warming oil while the second is distinctly cooling.

For another very effective massage oil mixture, take 8 ounces of Olive oil and scent it with ¼ ounce of essential oil of Sage. Sage is excellent for feet and legs, and can be added to bath water, hot foot soaks, or oils for massage.

TWISTS AND SPRAINS

One injury that I am thoroughly familiar with is the twisted knee. Although I have never played football or soccer or any other rough sport, I have been involved in several automobile accidents. They always seem to involve the knees and neck, whiplash in the latter and cracked kneecaps after bashing against the dashboard in the former. Once I had a skiing accident in which both legs rotated at the knee joint—my body pointing downhill while my feet pointed uphill. These injuries have been treated in various ways through the years—the most current knee injury having had the most effective treatment.

After the auto accident in which my knees were smashed against the dashboard I had difficulty walking up and down stairs. For two weeks after the accident stairs were navigated only with the greatest difficulty. I actually had to walk backward down stairs because of the pain. After the accident I was told by doctors that nothing could be done outside of surgery and massage therapy. I then determined to prescribe my own treatments. I spent nearly a year going to a massage therapist for weekly treatments. I found that hot and cold herbal soaks were very effective against the discomfort after a long walk or any exercise. Jogging was impossible, as were aerobics, although very-low-impact aerobics helped. Since I was no longer exercising with any regularity, I gained 20 pounds, which increased the burden on my knees. I should have started acupuncture treatments immediately after the injury but unfortunately I waited for a year. The acupuncture was painful but needn't have been; it does depend on the acupuncturist. After only 5 treatments I found that I was able to get up to a slow run. The treatments were very painful, and would have been ever so much more effective had I started them sooner. After a year, I was jogging and able to walk for some distance without much discomfort.

In any sort of injury involving a limb it is important to keep exercising—but go easy. If it's painful don't continue. Even exercising the limb opposite the one that is injured helps strengthen the injured limb. No one really understands why this is so but I believe it is a question of balance. The body wants to keep both sides in balance. If your left leg is in a cast, you can exercise the left moderately and the right vigorously. This keeps the injured side from wasting away.

Another treatment that is extremely effective in getting injured knees back in shape is a hot and cold herbal soak.

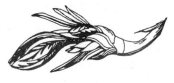

HOT AND COLD SOAKS FOR INJURIES

Use 1 ounce of Nettle herb, ½ ounce of Comfrey root, and ½ ounce of Peppermint or Sage. Use Nettle, Comfrey, and Sage for the hot infusion, and Nettle, Comfrey, and Peppermint for the cold soak. Use about 1 ounce total of mixed herbs for each mixture. This mixture and the watery infusion can be reused several times. Make the 2 infusions in the usual way, putting the cold one (with Peppermint) into the fridge. When needed, heat up your hot infusion until barely tolerable and soak the injury. While soaking in the hot, add ice to the other to chill it.

Soak in the hot infusion for at least 3 minutes, or use the herbs as a poultice and the liquid as a compress to warm the injured area. Then soak in the cold herbs or use cold compresses for at least 1 minute. Alternate the hot and cold for at least 20 minutes 3 times per day. You should feel a pleasant, soothing tingle, followed by loss of pain.

This treatment can be used for tennis elbow, knee injuries, twisted ankles, bursitis, and so on. Poultices are also very effective and either of the following two herbal mixtures seem to work extremely well:

Formula 1:   equal parts of Comfrey root, Rosemary, and Sage (cut and sifted or powder)

Formula 2:   equal parts of Comfrey root, Yarrow, Violet, and Pennyroyal (cut and sifted or powder)

In a shallow pan or dish, pour just enough boiling water over the herbs to thoroughly wet them without leaving a puddle. Apply the hot, wet herbs directly to the hurt. Cover with a cloth wrung out in very hot water. This is called a poultice. Cover with a plastic bag and then with a thick piece of wool or felt. Keep the heat in as long as possible. When the inner cloth cools, replace it with another hot one. Repeat for 15–30 minutes. Follow this with a *gentle* massage, using the general massage oil already recommended, and 85 percent DMSO if you have it. Please rest your injury for as long as possible until it heals. In summary, remember that injured joints need massage, hot and cold herbal soaks, acupuncture, exercise, and DMSO.

OTHER INJURIES

All the preceding formulas can be used for joggers or runners. Another problem that may occur sometimes after running is that blood may be passed with the urine. This occurs in men because the bladder hits against the prostate while they jog or run. Men should take the precaution of emptying their bladder before a run. Women do not have this problem; if they bleed when they run they should consult a sports-minded health practitioner.

Herbs such as King's Fern help back-related injuries. Use the gel as a back rub. Sage and Camomile seem to work especially

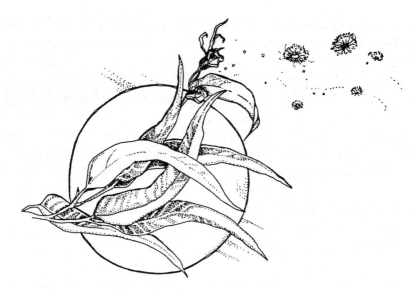

well in massage oils and herbal baths. Add these herbs to any of the preceding recipes for oils, baths, and soaks. Back injuries respond especially well to the combination of rest, then massage with oils, hot and cold showers (3 minutes hot and 1 minute cold, repeat 3 times for a total of 12 minutes), acupuncture treatments, and DMSO.

For better circulation infuse the various herbs listed for massage oils in alcohol to make an herbal alcohol rub. Add 1 ounce of mixed herbs to 2 cups rubbing alcohol and let steep for 10 days, shaking the container daily. Then strain the alcohol through a muslin or silk cloth, bottle the tincture, and rub it on weary, tired muscles to stimulate blood circulation.

If you overextend yourself, you may get nauseated and even vomit. Peppermint tea, excellent for nausea, and Ginger tea, recommended for stomachache or vomiting, or a single drop of oil of Peppermint in a half glass of water are all excellent to relax the stomach. They should all be sipped continually for about 30 minutes for best results. Peppermint tea or oil in water also works to alleviate car or motion sickness. Even your pets can take it, although the homeopathic Peppermint remedies seem more suitable for pets and babies. You can also use Camomile and Gentian tea as a remedy for nausea and the headaches that athletes sometimes get after strenuous performances and workouts.

For fears and stage fright before an athletic contest the best herbs are teas made of Camomile, Rose hips, Parsley, Alfalfa, Thyme, Rosemary, Mint, Lemon Verbena, Lemon peel, and Lemon Balm. These can be taken freely day or night before athletic activity. They have the ability to calm, even to strengthen and stimulate. These qualities may sound contradictory. But Rosemary, for instance, can stimulate the mind even while it balances the muscular system. Herbs often have these seemingly contradictory abilities. Remember that they are both foods and tonics, and they contain vitamins and minerals, and maybe this diversity of qualities will help explain their magic.

Lemon Verbena, Lemon peel and Lemon Balm are mildly sedative. Use a strong infusion an hour or two before bedtime the night before an athletic event to lull you to sleep. These herbs will not leave you feeling groggy or dull in the morning.

To clear up your eyesight before an athletic event use eyewashes or compresses of Linden flowers, Camomile flowers, Fennel seed, and Comfrey root. Other good eyewashes are mentioned in both the "First-Aid" and "Home Remedy" chapters. Compresses are especially effective if you use them while lying on a slant board; 18 inches off the floor is just about right.

Many reactions sportsmen get are specific to their sport, such as the cold hands of the early morning duck shoot, the sore and aching thighs and stiff rear end of a long-distance bicycle rider, the sore wrists of a bowler, or the aching feet of a fisherman. These aches and pains are all manifestations of the same general muscular problems—overuse or unaccustomed use. Use a loofah, a horsehair and hemp strap, or an Aloe fiber strap before or after excessive physical exercise to stimulate circulation. Take a warm herbal bath using herbs like Nettle for stimulation, Rosemary and Lavender for aching muscles, and Comfrey for healing. Then rub yourself briskly all over using the straps or brushes, massaging from the toes up toward the nose, and from the nose down toward the toes. After you bathe, get or give yourself a good massage using any of the herbal mixtures already described or a simple massage oil made of 8 ounces of vegetable oil scented with ¼ ounce essential oil of Rosemary or Sage. Sage is especially good for the feet and Rosemary for the long muscles of your legs and arms.

DIET

Remember that muscle spasms and pain can result from inadequate nutrition and mineral or vitamin deficiencies. If your spasms are caused by the former try drinking cold teas, especially from those herbs that contain silica, such as Horsetail and Oatstraw, and calcium herbs such as Comfrey, Borage, Chickweed, or Dandelion. Muscle spasms respond particularly well to Chaparral, which is better known as Creosote Bush, and to Thyme. Peppermint tea is also effective. If the spasms and pain are a result of vitamin and mineral deficiencies, step up your intake of calcium (as bonemeal or dolomite) and the B vitamins, especially with the use of brewer's yeast and Wheat germ. Magnesium is known to help muscle spasms, as are B_6, biotin, and pantothenic acid. Take plenty of bee pollen, vitamin C, and nucleic acids. The last 2 increase one's resistance to cold. All 3 improve the condition of the entire body.

So get into condition, train yourself carefully, eat plenty of wholesome basic foods with vitamin, mineral, and herbal supplements, and if you get muscle aches or spasms use the good herbs as directed.

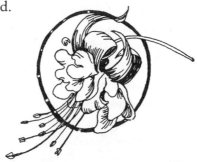

10

...

Herbal and Homeopathic First Aid

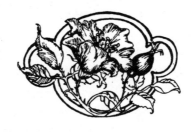

When I was a Girl Scout our motto was to always "be prepared"—to be ready for any situation. This attitude is most appropriate for the person who is traveling or vacationing, for the parent taking care of children, or the outdoors person. "Little" emergencies happen to all of us at one time or another.

As a Scout I began to carry a Swiss Army knife containing multiple tools that served a variety of purposes. When I was 10 the knife came in handy for digging holes in the ground and planting seedlings; as a grownup I use the same type of knife to cut Apples in half, to dissect unwary creatures for the edification and education of my nature class, or, sterilized, to open a nasty, infected wound or to open my bottle of wine when picnicking. I have used tweezers to pluck ungrateful hairs from my one eyebrow or nasty splinters from a finger. The knife is still an essential item in my first-aid kit, and a first-aid kit is essential to first aid.

THE HERBAL FIRST-AID KIT

Emergencies occur, from bruising to falling to eye irritations that need instant attention. One cannot wait 30 minutes to cook up an infusion or make a poultice and then wait until they can be used. A first-aid kit must be instantly accessible, the contents instantly usable. Also, a first-aid kit should not contain harmful ingredients. You will need only a small basket (1 foot by 1 foot by 4 inches) to carry everything a household needs for protection. With a little judicious trimming this can be reduced to half the size and be useful as a first-aid kit for the car. A further reduction of ingredients and you can carry your kit in your backpack for first aid on the trail.

I have experimented with and put together first-aid kits for years and find that the items in the following list are the most useful. Those marked T make up the traveling kit; those marked BP make up the backpacking and hiking kit; all are used in the home kit.

WHAT TO HAVE AVAILABLE IN YOUR FIRST-AID KIT

HERBAL SUPPLIES
Aloe vera gel/Comfrey root gel—2 ounces
Bruise Juice, a medicated oil—4 ounces (T, BP)
Calendula cream—1–2 ounce tube
Camomile, homeopathic tablets, 30x—small vial (T, BP)
Cayenne powder—1-oz plastic bottle (T)
Comfrey root, powder, and cut pieces—1 ounce each (T, BP)
Fennel seeds, whole—1 ounce (T)
Garlic oil perles—2-oz container (T, BP)
Goldenseal powder—1-oz plastic bottle
Ipecac syrup—comes prepackaged

Oils, essential
   Clove—½ oz
   Eucalyptus—1 oz
   Peppermint—½ oz (T)
   Rosemary—1 oz
Olive oil—4 oz
Papaya leaf tea bags—1 package
Salve, your favorite brand or homemade
Swiss Kriss—1 small bottle tablets (BP)
Tantra tabs—1 small box or bag (BP)
Tinctures
   Arnica—1-oz bottle (BP)
   Echinacea—1-oz bottle
   Goldenseal—1-oz bottle (BP)

NONHERBAL SUPPLIES

Antihistamine—1 small (4 oz) bottle (T)
Charcoal, activated—1 small bottle capsules (T, BP)
Chlorophyll—2-oz bottle
Clay—1-lb box (T)
DMSO (dimethylsulfoxide)—1-oz bottle (T, BP)
Green soap—4-oz bottle
Honey—2-oz container (BP)
Hydrogen peroxide—4-oz bottle (T)
Lecithin—1 small bottle (2-oz)
Vitamin E—1 small container (T, BP)

EQUIPMENT

Band-Aids in assorted sizes—1 box (T, BP)
Cotton—1 small roll (T)
Ear syringe—child size
Gauze pads—1 box
Gauze strips or muslin—tear them yourself
Hot water bottle with douche attachment
Magnifying glass—10x (T, BP)
Matches in waterproof case, use wooden matches (T, BP)

Moleskin—1 small package (T, BP)
Safety pins, assorted sizes—1 small container (T, BP)
Snakebite kit—comes prepackaged (T, BP)
Tampons—6 (T, BP)
Thermometer, anal type
Swiss Army knife with knife, scissors, tweezers, magnifying glass (T, BP)
Vaporizer, hot-air type, comes with a well for the addition of oils, or Aroma-Vera diffusor
Pen and note pad

SOURCES OF SUPPLIES

I have found mail order to be the most efficient way to get the ingredients I need for a first-aid kit. An herb store, a health food store, and a pharmacy yield items unobtainable by mail order.

The Herbal Bodyworks: 219 A Carl Street, San Francisco, CA 94117.
Catalog is $1 and will supply Bruise Juice, Aloe and Comfrey gel, Olive oil, clay, hand cream, and essential oils.

Weleda, Inc.: 30 South Main Street, Spring Valley, NY 10977.
Carries Calendula cream, salves, and excellent baby care products.

Aroma-Vera, P.O. Box 3609, Culver City, CA 90231.
Carries quality essential oils and books.

Boericke & Tafel, Inc.: 1011 Arch Street, Philadelphia, PA 19107.
Carries all homeopathic supplies, tablets, grains, creams, oils, succi, and lotions.

HERBAL FIRST-AID TREATMENTS

Anger: Camomile, 2–3 homeopathic tablets immediately. Repeat after 30 minutes.

Athlete's Foot: Dust with Goldenseal and Comfrey root powders during the day and wash with tincture of Goldenseal and Echinacea before bed.

Bee Stings: Poultice with Papaya leaf tea, then apply gel or cream or salve or Poultice (or both) with clay, then apply a mixture of DMSO and a dab of Goldenseal.

Blisters: Apply DSMO immediately, cover with moleskin. Apply paste of DMSO and Goldenseal and apply moleskin.

Bowel Distress: Take activated charcoal and Papaya leaf tea. For diarrhea or dysentery, take activated charcoal, 2–3 tablets, Papaya leaf tea with teaspoons of Chlorophyll every hour. For constipation, drink water, ¼ cup Olive oil and before bed take 2–3 Swiss Kriss tablets.

Bruises, Sprains: Apply cold immediately, then Bruise Juice and Arnica tincture or Arnica tincture and DMSO in a ratio of 1:1.

Coldness: Massage with Rosemary oil mixed with Olive oil; sprinkle area with Cayenne; take ½ teaspoon Cayenne at 2-hour intervals.

Colds and Fevers: Take 3 perles of Garlic every 4 hours plus ½ teasspoon Cayenne; vaporize as much as possible with Eucalyptus/Peppermint/Rosemary oil using a mixture of 2:1:1.

Crushed Fingers and Toes: Take tincture of Arnica in water, 25 drops every 15 minutes; apply a dressing of Arnica and Comfrey root.

Cuts, Scratches: Wash with green soap, apply a dilute tincture of Goldenseal and if large close edges with a butterfly Band-Aid.

Earaches: Wash out with warm Comfrey root infusion, squeeze oil from Garlic perles into ear every 4 hours, take Camomile tablets.

Embedded Objects: Clean area with warm water or Comfrey root water, remove object with tweezers.

Exhaustion: Rest if possible and take Camomile tablets until recovery is complete; or if you need to wake up, take 1 Tantra tab every 2–4 hours.

Eyes—Irritated or Red: Wash with infusion of Comfrey root and Fennel seed every hour until relieved.

Frostbite: Swab area with a solution of 90 percent DMSO with a few drops of Rosemary oil. Swab area every few hours until it is normal.

Headache: Rub temples with drop of Rosemary oil; take 1 drop mixed with ½ glass water internally.

Infected Wounds: Wash with green soap; apply continual poultices of clay until open and draining and then dust with Goldenseal powder.

Insect Bites: Wash with green soap; apply poultice of clay, clean and dust with clay or apply chlorophyll.

Insomnia: Take Camomile homeopathic, 3 tablets every 20 minutes until asleep.

Jet Lag: Take Camomile homeopathic, 2–3 tablets and alternate with dilute Arnica tincture, 25 drops in ½ glass of water.

Nosebleed: Lie down, apply compress of water and Rosemary oil on head and pinch nostrils until bleeding stops; take 10 drops tincture Arnica in ½ glass water.

Poison: Take Ipecac as directed.

Poison Oak or Ivy: Wash with green soap and cool water; apply paste of clay and Goldenseal powder.

Sore Muscles: Rub and massage area with a mixture of Rosemary oil and Olive oil in a ratio of 1:5.

Sprains: Apply cold if possible, then a mixture of DMSO and Bruise Juice in a ratio of 5:1.

Stomachache: Take capsules of activated charcoal and drink Papaya leaf tea; take 2 drops Peppermint oil in ½ glass water.

Sunburn: Cool the area with compresses of cold water and Comfrey root; apply Aloe gel or vitamin E every 2 hours.

Sunstroke, Heatstroke: Lie down and cool body with cold compresses of water with a drop of Peppermint oil added; or sit in a cool-water bath.

Toothache: Put a drop of Clove oil on a piece of cotton and insert into the aching tooth; take 2–3 capsules of Garlic oil internally every 4 hours.

Tooth, Infected: Wash mouth out with chlorophyll every 2 hours; at night apply a paste of charcoal to the infected area and hold in place with a piece of cotton.

Vomiting: Mix 2 drops oil of Peppermint with ½ cup of water and sip continually; repeat when necessary.

AN HERBAL FIRST-AID TALE

By way of wrapping up this section, and as a way of letting you in on one of my herbal first-aid cure-alls, I'd like to tell you about an incident that happened in my own life. It is an herbal first-aid tale, and involves a dire accident, but not to worry—all herbal tales have happy endings.

During my last battle with raiding raccoons, I was painting my patio bricks with an oil of Capsicum paste, a pure form of Cayenne that is supposed to keep the critters away. While I was doing this a bit of the oil splashed onto my face and into my eyes. I was immediately blinded. I stumbled into the house, remembering that many of the old herbalists had used ground Cayenne pepper as an aromatic stimulant on cuts, including around the eyes. Hoping that this pure oil of Capsicum would be as ultimately harmless as the ground pepper, I nonetheless began flushing my throbbing, burning eyes and face with water while I dialed the emergency operator to connect me with Poison Control Center. The people at the Poison Control told me to continue flushing with water while they looked up the toxicity of this extremely concentrated oil. While they were off the line, which was about 15 minutes, I applied a number of my usual first-aid remedies hoping to cool my skin and help my eyes. All this time I was totally unable to see out of the right eye, and the left wasn't much better. I applied yogurt, which did not work, then baking soda, which also did not work, then Bruise Juice, then Mullein oil to my skin. None of these remedies had the slightest effect on my condition. Finally, I stumbled to the refrigerator to get my Fennel/Comfrey First-Aid Remedy and began to wash my eyes with this cold solution using an eyecup. Immediately, the pain ceased in both my eyes and on my face. My eyes were of course extremely bloodshot. Cayenne pepper is a stimulant and rubefacient and is often used directly on hemorrhaging wounds to stop the bleeding. The effects of the pure oil of a substance can be quite different from the effects of the herb itself (see Chapter 12). I also took a homeopathic remedy called Calms Forte containing plant extracts of Passion Flower (Passiflora), Camomile (Chamomilla), Oats (Avena), Hops (Humulus lupulus), and Calcarea Phosphorica, Ferrum Phosphoricum, Kali Phosphoricum, Magnesia Phosphorica, and Natrum Phosphoricum. This remedy is extremely good for calming adults as well as children, is quite safe to take, and is also used for insomnia and nervous tension.

After 15 minutes, the Poison Control Center called back to tell me that the active ingredient of the oil, capsaicin, is excruciatingly painful (which I certainly was well aware of) but not harmful.

The fantastic Fennel/Comfrey First-Aid remedy has already been mentioned but I've saved the formula till now because it's so special. It is very easy to make and should be kept in the fridge at all times. There it stays cold and so has double value for burns or sunburn. It can be used both internally and externally.

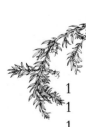

JEANNE ROSE'S FANTASTIC FENNEL/ COMFREY REMEDY

1	T Fennel seed, whole
1	T Comfrey root, either fresh or dried pieces
1	cup water

Bring everything to a boil in a small, covered enamel pan. Reduce heat and simmer for about 3 minutes. Turn off heat and let cool on the stove. When cool enough to handle, strain through a piece of silk or double thickness of cheesecloth into a clean container. Store in the refrigerator. Make a fresh solution every 3–4 days, using the old one as a fertilizer for house plants or drinking it as an aid to good digestion.

HOMEOPATHIC FIRST AID

It is startling to learn that homeopaths use Stinging Nettle *(Urtica urens)* to treat people with first- or second-degree burns. Of course, a homeopath would not recommend actually touching a Stinging Nettle plant to the burned area. Instead, a homeopath would give a specially prepared, nontoxic dose of Stinging Nettle. Although Stinging Nettle causes a burn when one is exposed to it in toxic dose, it also helps *heal* burns when taken in a small, nontoxic dose.

The basic principle of homeopathic medicine is that a small dose of a substance will help cure that which it causes in overdose. For instance, Alliumcepa, from Onions, which make you tear when cut, is used as a homeopathic remedy for head colds and watery nasal secretions. Although this principle may be a bit confusing at first, it actually makes a lot of sense. Modern physiology and biology are confirming a basic premise of homeopathy, that symptoms are efforts of the organism to adapt to stress. Symptoms are therefore understood as the way the "bodymind" is trying, although not always successfully, to re-establish homeostasis, or balance. Since symptoms are the best efforts of the organism to attempt to heal itself, it is better to aid and stimulate the body's defense processes than to treat or sup-press specific symptoms.

Homeopaths, like doctors using conventional immunizations and allergy treatments, stimulate the defense system by giving small doses of what causes a condition in order to create a response from the immune system. Homeopathic medicines, however, are distinctively different from immunizations and allergy treatments, in that the homeopathic medicines are tai-lored to an individual's specific needs, are given in much smaller and less toxic doses, and are used for both prevention and treatment of a person.

Homeopathic medicine developed much of its popularity in the United States and Europe because of its success in treating people with cholera, scarlet fever, yellow fever, and other infec-tious diseases that were ravaging populations. More recently homeopathic medicine has developed a reputation of success-fully treating people with various chronic complaints. What many people do not know about homeopathy is that it also provides many valuable medicines in treating people who suffer from accidents and injuries. When these medicines are used in conjunction with conventional first-aid procedures, the risk of long-term damage from an injury can be significantly decreased and the healing process can be noticeably enhanced.

One must study homeopathic medicine for many years to learn how to prescribe the correct medicine for people with chronic conditions. One can, however, learn to use the medi-cines for first aid very easily. Whereas treatment of a person's acute or chronic disease requires strict examination of and ad-justment of the treatment to the person's total physical and psychological state, treatment for accidents and injuries does not require such individualized prescription. The reason for this difference is that people with acute or chronic diseases have distinct or subtly different symptoms and causes of their condition, and thus each needs a different medicine to begin the curative process. People with injuries tend to experience very similar symptoms and usually need a similar metabolic stimulus to heal their complaint. Basically, when different people cut themselves, get burned, break a leg, or injure themselves in some other way, they all tend to need a similar stimulus to heal their injury.

The medicines in the following list are used to treat people in first-aid situations. There are other homeopathic medicines that can also used, but these are the most commonly used medicines for the conditions described.

Homeopaths use the Latin names for their medicines, since they need a universally recognized nomenclature to allow them to converse with homeopaths throughout the world. In the following catalog the Latin names are given first and the common name follows in parentheses. After this listing you will find some helpful information on the dosage, administration, and storage of homeopathic first-aid medicines, most of which you should be able to find in a good health-food store.

Arnica (Mountain Daisy). Arnica is mentioned first because it is a medicine *par excellence* for the shock or trauma of any injury. It is necessary to treat an injured person for shock first unless the injury is very mild or the person is bleeding so profusely that stopping the bleeding should be attended to immediately. Since Arnica is the first medicine prescribed in numerous types of injuries, it is the most common medicine used in first aid. It helps reduce shock, relieve pain, diminish swelling, and begin healing. It is also an excellent medicine before or after surgery, since the body experiences a state of shock from these medical procedures. It is also used before and after dental surgery and before, during, and after labor to help mother and infant deal with the shock and stress of birth.

Hypericum (St.-John's-Wort). Hypericum tincture is recommended as an external application in treating deep cuts, since it helps heal internal structures as well as the skin. It also has the ability to close open wounds and thus sometimes prevents the need for stitches. Hypericum is also used for septic (infected) wounds (Calendula, in comparison, is primarily good for clean, uninfected cuts). Hypericum tincture, like other external applications that have an alcoholic base, should be diluted before application. Hypericum compress is an excellent medicine for injuries to nerves or to injured parts of the body that are richly supplied with nerves (fingers, toes, the spine). Generally, such injuries have sharp or shooting pain, or both, and the injured part is very sensitive to touch. Hypericum is also good for old injuries to nerves that still bother a person.

Urtica Urens (Stinging Nettle). As you might have predicted from the law of similars, Urtica Urens is the medicine of choice for burns (Stinging Nettle, as you may know, causes a burn upon contact with the spine of the plant). Urtica Urens in external application is also helpful in diminishing the pain of the burn and in promoting healing. Such application should be diluted approximately 1 part of Urtica Urens with 10 parts water.

Ledum (Marsh Tea). Ledum is the best medicine for a puncture wound, whether it be from a needle, from a nail, or a septic scratch. Deep punctures or punctures from rusty nails should receive medical attention, but this should not delay you from taking Ledum, which has no side effects and which can be helpful in healing wounds and preventing tetanus. Ledum is also commonly prescribed for insect stings and animal bites. It is also applicable to people with severe bruising (black eyes or blows from firm objects), especially if the affected part feels cold and yet feels relieved by cold applications.

Rhus Tox (Poison Ivy). Although some people cringe when they even hear someone mention Poison Ivy, it is an often-prescribed homeopathic medicine (in *nontoxic* homeopathically prepared doses) for a certain type of skin condition as well as for numerous other conditions that homeopaths have found it causes in overdose. One of the conditions it causes in overdose is the rupturing of ligaments and tendons. Because of this, it is the most common medicine prescribed for sprains and strains, especially the type of sprain or strain that is worse upon initial motion but better upon continued motion. It is also a medicine given for dislocated joints. Arnica is another medicine to consider for dislocations.

Ruta (Rue). Ruta is the medicine given for severe sprains when the person has a torn or wrenched tendon, split ligament, or bruises periosteum (bone covering). It is also the most common medicine prescribed for recent or old injuries to the knee or elbow, and it is prescribed for tennis elbow.

Symphytum (Comfrey). Homeopaths, like herbalists, like Symphytum for fractures. Homeopaths, however, give their medicine in potentized dose, while herbalists use it in teas and poultices. Although one must go to a physician to have the fracture reset and placed in a cast, Symphytum will relieve pain and promote rapid healing of the fracture. Besides its application in fractures, Symphytum is a great medicine for injuries to the eyeball, the bones around the eye, and the cheekbones.

Some homeopathic medicines are for *external application* only.

Calendula (Marigold). Calendula tincture (in an alcohol base), Calendula oil (in a mineral oil base) and Calendula cerate (ointments with wax) are all invaluable external applications in treating cuts and abrasions. Calendula is known to have antiseptic properties because of its organic iodine content. Calendula helps stop bleeding, inhibit infection, and promote granulation of tissues to heal wounds and burns. Calendula tincture should not be applied directly on a cut, since its alcoholic content causes stinging pain. It's best to dilute this tincture with a little water. If you'd like to avoid this effort, you can instead directly apply Calendula oil or Calendula cerate. (*Note:* Calendula works so rapidly in healing the skin that it is not recommended for use in deep cuts. In deep cuts Calendula sometimes can close and heal the outside skin while the tissue under the skin is not yet completely healed.)

GENERAL RULES FOR DETERMINING DOSAGE

People who are beginners in homeopathy should primarily use the 6x (sixth potency) or 30x. Only homeopathic practitioners who have a great deal of knowledge of homeopathy should use the higher potencies (200x, 1000x, and higher). Homeopathic medicines are more powerful the more they are potentized. Higher potencies thus should be used with great care.

Homeopaths have found that injured people tend to need more frequent repetition of doses shortly after injury. One may need to prescribe a medicine every 30 to 60 minutes immediately after a severe injury. After a couple of hours, the frequency of doses can diminish to every other hour or every fourth hour, depending upon the severity of pain. Doses every 4 hours or 4 times a day are common when the person has a nonsevere injury. A person will generally not need to take a medicine for more than 2 to 4 days, except with fractures or severe sprains, for which 1 to 3 doses daily for 5 to 7 days are common.

A medicine should only be taken as long as the person experiences pain. Do *not* continue taking the medicine unless there are still symptoms. One risks taking an overdose of the medicine if one continues to take the medicine. *The basic idea is to take as little of the medicine as possible and yet enough to lessen pain and stimulate one's healing powers.* The more severe the condition, the more often will its repetition generally be necessary.

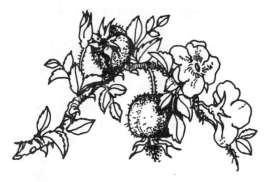

ADMINISTRATION OF THE MEDICINE

The medicine should be taken into a "clean mouth." Food, drink, tobacco, toothpaste, and other substances should not be put into the mouth for at least 15 minutes before or after the dose. It is generally best to place the medicine underneath the tongue.

Homeopaths have found that some substances can neutralize the effects of the medicines. Although there is some controversy over which substances are implicated, it is best to avoid the following substances for at least 48 hours after taking the final dose: coffee, camphorated products (including lip balm, counterirritant muscle-relaxing cremes, tiger's balm), teas (including herbal teas), mentholated products, cough drops, and mouthwash. Homeopaths will generally recommend that individuals who are being treated for a chronic condition avoid coffee and camphorated products for a longer period.

CARE AND STORAGE OF HOMEOPATHIC MEDICINES

Special handling and storage of the homeopathic medicines are needed in order to avoid contamination. When the medicines are correctly handled and stored, homeopaths have found that they can last for several generations. Since it is very difficult to determine if the medicines have been contaminated, one should take the following precautions to prevent problems:

- They should be kept away from strong light, from temperatures higher than 100 degrees, and from exposure to strong odors, such as camphor, menthol, mothballs, or perfumes.
- They should always be kept in the container in which they were supplied and never transferred to any other bottle that has contained other substances.
- They should be opened for administration of the medicine for the minimum time possible. One should be careful not to contaminate the cap or cork before replacement.
- It is important never to open more than 1 bottle at a time in a room. Failure to take this precaution can result in crosspotentization and spoiling of the medicines.
- If, by accident, more pills than the number specified in the prescribed dose are shaken out of the bottle, do not return them to the container; throw the excess away to avoid possible contamination.

If you would like to learn more about homeopathy, you can obtain a free list of homeopathic books and other information by sending a stamped, self-addressed envelope to Homeopathic Educational Services, 2124 Kittredge Street, Berkeley, CA 94704, or 5916 Chabot Crest, Oakland, CA.

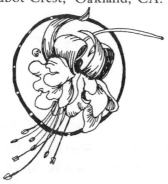

11

· · ·

Tips for Preparing Herbs as Cures

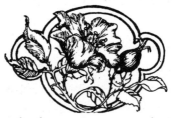

There are many methods one can use to administer herbal medicines and many modes of preparation. Each of these methods and preparations can be performed in many different ways, some of which I have described in other works. There is no best method. Twenty years ago, when I first started making herbal infusions, I used the standard directions that I had seen in many books: heat the teapot, put in ½ ounce to 1 ounce of herb, add 2 cups boiling water, and steep 10–20 minutes. Now my method of preparing an infusion is quite different and neither the original nor my modernized version is "better."

Tea (beverage). Warm pot, boil 1 cup water. Pour boiling water over approximately 1 tablespoon of herbs, cover, and *steep* 3–5 minutes. With more herbs and longer steeping this becomes an infusion and therefore more medicinal.

Tisane (also Barley Water or Ptisan). A nourishing decoction or infusion, which often has a slight medicinal quality, originally made from Barley. Now frequently used for a beverage tea made from flowers. Can also be defined as an infusion of herbs.

Infusion. An infusion usually involves the soft parts of the plant, such as the herb, leaf, or flower, 1 ounce of which is soaked or "infused" for 10–20 minutes in up to 1 quart of just-below-boiling (temperature) water. Simmer the herbs a moment or two and then infuse them.

Decoction. A decoction is usually made of the hard parts of the plant, such as the root, bark, or seed—the tougher parts. Put 1 ounce of herb and 20 ounces of water into a pot. Bring to a boil and simmer for 10–20 minutes or longer. Steep, strain, and drink. If making decoction from both hard and soft parts, boil the hard parts (such as the bark and seeds) and add the soft parts (such as the herb or flower) during the steeping cycle.

Ointment. A medicinal ointment is simply an herb crisped in lard, strained, cooled, and stored. This constitutes a "simple." Simmer 1 ounce of the herb in 4 ounces of lard (or Crisco, or whatever) in a nonmetal pot, preferably a double boiler, for 10–30 minutes. Strain and cool. Different simples may be mixed for different effects.

Cerate. Use a single herb or a mixture of herbs. The mixture of herbs depends on the effects desired. Cerates are also cosmetic creams. Simmer 1 ounce herbs in 8 ounces oil plus 1 ounce of wine until the wine is boiled off. Strain off the herbs, add ½ ounce solidifier (beeswax or lanolin), heat only until everything is incorporated, remove from heat, and beat with a wooden spoon or whisk until cool.

Plaster. A plaster is usually a macerated, bruised bunch of fresh hot herbs places between 2 sheets of muslin and applied to the aching or bruised area, or to the chest for respiratory problems. Causes increased circulation and sweating, which cleanses the system of impurities, lowers fever, and reduces swelling.

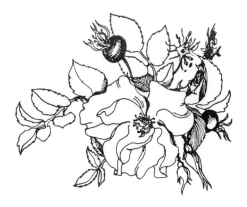

Poultice. Same as plaster, except the herbs are applied directly and a hot cloth wrapped around to keep them hot. Used to open a dirty sore or abscess.

Elixir. Infuse 4 ounces herbs in 4 ounces or more boiling water for 10 minutes or longer. Add 8 ounces 100-proof vodka. Strain off the herbs through a silk cloth and squeeze out the liquid completely. Set aside the squeezed herbs for other uses. You can also add a sweetener to the elixir (liquid) for taste. Honey will act as a natural preservative. Take a teaspoonful or so every hour like a cough syrup. A child should take a teaspoonful every 4 hours.

Mellite. 1 ounce herb, 20 ounces water. Boil 20 minutes. Strain and add 4 or more ounces of honey.

Syrup. 1 ounce herb, 20 ounces water, simmer 20 minutes. Strain and add 4–8 ounces sugar—to taste.

Tincture. Tinctures are very concentrated solutions that can be added to teas and infusions or diluted for use in cosmetic or medicinal preparations. They can be kept for long periods in a very small space. A tincture is a solution of medicinal substances in alcohol, prepared by maceration, digestion, or percolation. Herbs whose active ingredients have been extracted by alcohol are also called tinctures. The advantage of alcohol over water (as in a tea or infusion) is that alcohol dissolves some substances that are sparingly or not at all soluble in water. Another advantage is that alcohol is a preservative. The disadvantage, of course, is that if you need many herbs at the same time you may ingest too much alcohol.

The time-honored way of making tinctures is as follows: Start with 150-proof (60–80 percent) alcohol. I use vodka since it generally does not alter the taste of the herbal tincture. Originally, high-proof brandy was used, but brandy taste often does not mix well with herb taste.

Take about 4 ounces of your herb, root, bark, or seed and bruise, slice, or pulverize it. It is best to work with plants in the dry state, as tinctures made with freshly picked plants are not as good. Coarsely ground herbs are better than powdered because the powders often stick together and do not extract well. When making a tincture of several substances use the least soluble first, such as bark, then seed, then herb, and then flower; this allows the different substances to macerate for successively shorter lengths of time depending on their delicacy or lack of it.

Add 2 pints (4 cups) alcohol to the pulverized or coarsely ground herb. Two weeks is the usual amount of time to allow the herb and alcohol to commingle, though the time really depends on the substance. Flowers, for instance, take only a few days to soak (macerate) in the alcohol while barks may take several months. Shake or stir daily.

When the tincture has taken on the quality of the plant material (scent, color, vitality), strain carefully through several layers of cheesecloth or silk cloth, or press through a hydraulic press.

Store in small lightproof containers in a dark place. Note that the preceding directions are very general and that properly made tinctures are a result of careful work and judgment on the part of the maker. Each plant has its own characteristics—its own scent, time of extraction, and so forth. These must all be taken into account when making tinctures. Here are some examples:

A FLOWER TINCTURE

Put 2 ounces of freshly picked but half-dried flowers minus their calyx and green parts into a mortar, add ½ cup of 150-proof vodka or brandy, and mash and pulverize the mixture with a pestle. Pack the mixture into a container such as a glass bottle. Add 1½ cups of 150-proof vodka and stir thoroughly. Store in a cool, dark place for about a week. Stir the mixture every day. Strain carefully through silk and store in small light-proof bottles. You should have about 2 cups of tincture. If the mixture is not strong enough, go through the entire process, reusing the old (that is, the first-made) tincture, adding 2 more fresh ounces of flowers. You can call this Flower Tincture Times 2. Dose: 10 drops 3 times per day.

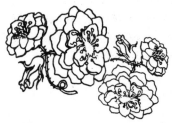

A BARK TINCTURE

Put 2 ounces dried, coarsely ground bark into a mortar and add ½ cup 150-proof vodka or brandy. Mash and pulverize with the pestle. Pack into a container and add 1½ cups more of the 150-proof alcohol. Stir thoroughly. Leave this to sit until the alcohol takes on the flavor and scent of the bark. Perfume tinctures of Clove and Cinnamon may take as long as 2 months. Stir every day. When the bark is exhausted (no flavor or scent left), if the tincture is still not strong enough, add more bark, repeating the process until the tincture is strong and full of color. Strain carefully through silk cloth and store in small lightproof containers. If the tincture is to be a perfume it may be used as is, or you can dilute it with oil or water to make a perfume oil or cologne. *Medicinal use:* up to 10 drops 3 times per day. *Cosmetic application:* diluted in oil or water and used as desired (externally).

A FLOWER AND BARK TINCTURE
(Rose and Cinnamon Perfume)

Put 2 ounces dried, coarsely ground bark into a mortar and add ½ cup of 150-proof alcohol, preferably vodka. Mash and pulverize with a pestle. Transfer to a lightproof container and add 1½ cups more alcohol. Stir thoroughly. Stir every day until the alcohol has taken on the scent and color of the bark. Now put 2 ounces highly perfumed flowers into a large mortar, add half of the bark tincture, and mash with the pestle. Transfer this back into the container and stir the contents thoroughly. Let sit for about a week, stirring the contents every day. Strain carefully through cheesecloth and put into small lightproof containers. *Medicinal dose:* up to 10 drops 3 times per day. *Cosmetic application:* Essential oil of the flower may be added as desired to the tincture to strengthen it, but if essential oil *is* added no more than 3 drops should be taken or applied at any time and no more than twice daily.

TINCTURE AURANTII
(Tincture of Orange Peel)

"Take of Bitter Orange Peel, cut small and bruised, two ounces; Proof Spirit one pint. Macerate for seven days in a closed vessel, with occasional agitation, then strain, press, and filter, and add sufficient Proof Spirit to make one pint." *(U.S. Dispensatory of the U.S.A.,* thirteenth edition, 1873). It is the peel of the Seville Orange that is referred to in this process. Only the outer part should be used; the inner, whitish portion is inert (insofar as scent goes, although it is very rich in bioflavonoids). The tincture of Orange peel is a welcome addition to infusions, decoctions, and mixtures. The dose is 1 or 2 fluidrams (1–2 teaspoons).

12

· · ·

Aromatherapy and Color Therapy

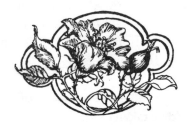

AROMATHERAPY

In his essays Francis Bacon wrote frequently on the scents of flowers and their effects. A passage in one of his essays makes an excellent introduction to the subject of aromatherapy:

> And because the breath of flowers is far sweeter in the air (where it comes and goes like the warbling of music) than in the hand, therefore nothing is more fit for that delight, than to know what be the flowers and plants that do best perfume the air. Roses, damask and red, are fast flowers of their smells; so that you may walk by a whole row of them, and find nothing of their sweetness; yea though it be in a mornings dew. Bays likewise yield no smell as they grow. Rosemary little; nor Sweet Marjoram. That which above all others yields the sweetest smell in the air, is the Violet, specially the White double Violet which comes twice a year; about the middle of April, and about Bartholomew-tide. Next to that is the Musk-Rose (flowering

in May/June). Then the Strawberry-leaves dying, with a most excellent cordial smell. Then the flower of the vines; it is a little dust, like the dust of a bent, which grows upon the cluster of the first coming forth. Then Sweet-brier (the Eglantine rose). Then Wall-flowers, which are very delightful to be set under a parlour or lower chamber window. Then Pinks and Gilliflowers, specially the matted pink and Clove Gilliflower. Then the flowers of the Lime-tree. Then the Honeysuckles, so they be somewhat afar off. Of Bean flowers I speak not, because they are field flowers. But those which perfume the air most delightfully, not passed by as the rest, but being trodden upon and crushed, are three; that is, Burnet, Wild-thyme, and Watermints. Therefore you are to set whole alleys of them, to have the pleasure when you walk or tread.

As spring approaches, the scents and aromas of little tree buds and flower buds waft through the air, tantalizing your nose with memories of times past. We know that the sense of smell is the most memoristic of the senses; the word *aromemories* describes the memories brought to the surface by aromas. Aromas affect the mind, of this we can be sure, but you can also rest assured that particular aromas applied in specific ways definitely affect the body. Aromatherapy is a way of treating mental and physical illness through the inhalation and application of volatile oils of plants; it also can be defined as combining the use of pure essential oils with pressure point therapy to treat illness. The following brief table will show the relationships between essential oils or essences of plants and how they act.

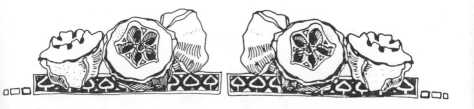

Classes of Essence	Includes the Oils From	Acts Upon	Causes	Used to Treat
Top notes	Flowers	The spirit	Stimulation and uplifting	Lethargy, melancholy, or lack of interest
Middle notes	Spices and herbs	Digestion and metabolism	Balance and tone	Inability to concentrate, blood pressure, and bodily functions
Base notes	Gums and woods	Mucous membranes and chronic conditions	Solidity and sedation	Nervousness, persons with erratic or flighty temperaments or conditions of long standing, or the elderly

Think f the *note* of a scent as a note in music: It indicates a single impression. The *top note* is the first scent impression of a fragrance. As designed by the perfumer, the top note is ephemeral and volatile. The *middle note* is the second stage in the development of a fragrance. What next hits your nose is what occurs between the top note and the base note, or that which bridges them. The *base note* is the final expression of the fragrance. Flowers generally have a volatile or ephemeral quality and almost always compose the top note in a combination scent, while herbs and spices are a bridge to the deeper and more lasting scents of gums and woods.

With the basic relationships shown in the table in mind, we must also know how and where to apply essential oils. There are several modes of application.

Direct inhalation of the odors. This generally affects the mind in a psychological way, although inhalation can also have direct physiological effect (for example, the inhalation of Eucalyptus oil from a steam bath or vaporizer to thin mucous secretions), and acts as an expectorant when your respiratory system is clogged.

Direct application of oils on acupuncture points using various forms of vigorous massage, such as Shiatsu, which has a physiological effect generally through the nervous system by way of the skin.

Indirect application of oils, by diluting them with vegetable oils or by extraction of essential oils derived from vegetable oils, used along with gentler forms of massage that aid the oil penetration and generally stimulate and relax to treat local problems.

Taking extremely *small doses of oil internally,* which has a direct physiological effect on organs and tissues.

The *application of essential oils derived from the original plant* in the form of herbal baths, herbal inhalations, facial steams, and so forth.

Aromatherapy has a rejuvenating and regenerating effect on the body. It is a modern method of natural treatment and can help in the rejuvenation and regeneration of the human body. It can help to improve physiological condition generally and render a person less vulnerable to illness. We know that this form of treatment has been in use for thousands of years. It is both an effective and an aesthetic therapy, and when properly applied has a tremendous influence in restoring health and vitality to the tissues while regulating capillary system activity and improving circulation.

Marguerite Maury, a magnificent proponent of aromatherapy as an art, felt that old age could be conquered through the use of the essential oils, and in fact wrote *The Secret of Life and Youth—Regeneration through Essential Oils* with that in mind.

HOW TO EXTRACT SCENT

There are many methods to "get" the scent out of a plant and these have been detailed in several books including my own *Herbal Body Book* and *Kitchen Cosmetics.* That great English herbalist Mrs. C. F. Leyel describes one method in her book

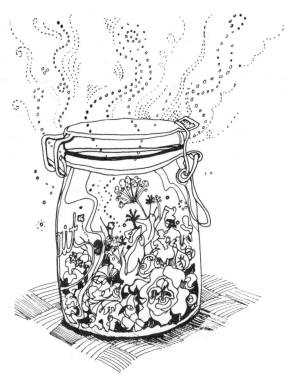

The Magic of Herbs, A Modern Book of Secrets: Fill a large jar three-quarters full of Olive oil, topping it off with the flowers of the Jasmine and any other sweet-smelling flowers. Small flowers should be chosen, and they should all be stripped of their stalks and leaves to leave room for as many flowers as possible. Leave them to macerate for 24 hours, then pour the contents of the whole jar into a black bag and squeeze the oil from it into another jar, to which more flowers must be added and the process repeated for 20 days, according to the strength required. Then the oil must be mixed with an equal quantity of strong, deodorized alcohol, and the mixture must be shaken every day for a fortnight. By that time the spirit should be highly scented, and it can be poured off, looking clear and bright.

I should add to this recipe that the Olive oil should be the best-quality Italian oil that you can obtain; California Olive oil will not do: It's too "green" smelling. If you want your end result to be one flower then you must start and finish with the same flower since this recipe yields a perfume rather than an extract or infused oil. The alcohol should also be the kind you can drink if you intend to take this internally. The same applies if you are using it externally in massage or as a perfume. A good quality vodka is fine and in some states pure alcohol is available through laboratories and some package stores. If you do take it internally, realize that the end result is a highly concentrated product representing an enormous number of flowers and should be taken like Bach flower remedies, that is, only *a few drops* of the tincted oils in a bit of water.

There is an art to the extraction of scent from flowers. This art is probably much older than distillation. Distillation is generally used for the green herbs but home extraction methods will yield a good quality of tincted or infused oil if care is taken.

WHEN TO APPLY SCENT

Life energy flows through the body, cyclically, along paths called meridians. Each meridian has a time during each day when it may most beneficially be treated. The lung time or lung meridian is 3:00 to 5:00 A.M., and this is indeed the best time to use aromas therapeutically, but if this seems a little early for you, remember that the morning is better than any other time for aroma massage or aromatherapy.

AROMATHERAPY MASSAGE

The deep thumb pressures of Shiatsu; the pressure of deep tissue massage intended to reach nerves, ligaments and tendons; the soft tissue work called Swedish massage; and the slow, gentle, rhythmic movement of effleurage massage are all used in aromatherapy massage. The total effect should be harmonious, not jarring in any way. Even deep tissue work should be done gently rather than vigorously. The purpose of aromatherapy massage is to aid in the penetration of the oil, to stimulate the body or to relax the body, to treat local problems, to treat via nerve supply, reflexes, or meridians.

Get a chart showing the spinal nerve roots and you will notice that there are 5 distinct sets of vertebrae. Have a friend massage along the indentation on either side of the spine. If you are a beginner just rub gently up and down this spinal gutter in small circular motions using the thumbs. Massage to loosen the area, then apply essential oil or infused oil and massage again. Specific oils can be used on specific nerve roots to affect specific organs or certain general oils can be applied along the entire body for a relaxing or stimulating effect. Geranium oil is especially useful along the cervical vertebrae and affects the skin. Bergamot-infused oil is good along the entire dorsal vertebrae as this oil (infused from the rind of a citrus fruit) has an antispasmodic effect on all the internal organs. Fennel oil is useful along the upper lumbar vertebrae as it affects the intestine (especially the large intestine) to release trapped gas and in general act as a tonic. Jasmine oil is very relaxing for the entire body and especially useful along the lumbar vertebrae where it can act to relieve certain sexual difficulties. A massage using oil of Rose is in general balancing, while Peppermint-infused oil is stimulating to the entire body and especially useful along the cervical vertebrae to reduce brain fatigue or headache.

SPECIFIC OIL QUALITIES

Basil oil is extracted from the herb and is especially useful for respiratory difficulties such as bronchitis. It acts as an antispasmodic and expectorant. It is also useful for nervous tension and headache. A useful mixture to detoxify the nose and relieve stuffy sinus is 1 part Juniper Berry oil to 2 parts each of Eucalyptus oil and Basil oil. Add 12–15 drops of this mixture to the well of a hot vaporizer and allow the warm, moist air to flow in an enclosed room. Eucalyptus oil extracted from the leaf is considered more of a yin oil, while Basil oil is yang. Eucalyptus oil has an antiseptic, deodorant, expectorant effect and works especially well on the respiratory system to relieve thick mucous secretions and fevers.

Fennel oil extracted from the fruit is considered a yang oil and is useful for digestive disturbances or flatulence. It is also an excellent diuretic and helps to heal the bladder and clear the urine. A good way to take the oil is to place a drop or 2 of it in a half-glass of water and drink in the morning before breakfast. It's also useful to relieve morning sickness. Juniper Berry oil, a yang oil extracted from the fruit, acts on the skin, digestion, urinary tract, blood, and nerves. Along with Sandalwood it is one of the classic diuretics and remedies for urinary tract infections.

A short list of problems that can be treated with essential oils: acne (Bergamot, Lavender, Sandalwood); allergies (Camomile, Mullein); asthma (Eucalyptus, Marjoram, Lavender); colds and bronchitis (Basil, Eucalyptus, Lavender, Rosemary); earache (Mullein, Black Pepper); fevers (Peppermint, Black Pepper); headache (Moroccan Jasmine); hysteria (Basil, Camomile, Marjoram, Neroli, Jasmine, Rose); mental exhaustion (Peppermint, Rosemary, Basil); obesity (Fennel, Juniper, Patchouli); rejuvenation (Rose, Melissa, Neroli, Jasmine, Patchouli); skin care (all oils, the specific one depends on the problem); painful cramps in pregnancy (Carnation). Other problems and oils are listed in *The Herbal Body Book*.

This is an extremely brief description of aromatherapy and its uses. The use of aromata is just one part of the path that leads to total health and beauty. Remember that good nutrition, exercise, clean water, and clean air form the rest of the prescription.

An excellent source on the healing arts, which includes a bit about aromatherapy (besides my *Herbal Body Book*) is *Stay Young* by Ivan Popov. He details the way to a happy, long life as follows: 1) have a happy marital and sexual situation; 2) there should *not* be a great abundance of food eaten; 3) clean fresh air, clean fresh water, and clean fresh natural food should be taken;

and 4) food should emphasize fresh fruits and vegetables and the fermented foods such as sauerkraut, kefir, and yogurt, and deemphasize meat. Both *Stay Young* and *The Herbal Body Book* were published by Grosset and Dunlap and are available through The Putnam Publishing Group, and they are available in paperback. Another book to note, one which was of great help to me in compiling the following calendar, "Color Therapy and Aromatherapy Throughout the Year," is *The Art of Aroma Therapy*, by Robert B. Tisserand.

Oils must be natural to be effective. That is, they must actually be extracted from a plant; synthetic oils are not acceptable in aromatherapy. There are several sources of really good pure essential oils. You will have to investigate the various herb stores and health food stores in your area (Chapter 6 in *The Herbal Body Book* lists mail-order sources) or get them from Aroma-Vera in Culver City, CA or Herbal Bodywork (address on page 173).

COLOR THERAPY

The use of color to influence human health is called color therapy. This type of therapy has been in use for hundreds of years. At this point it may be more or less an aesthetic or ethereal form of treatment. Nevertheless, it works. Medicine is very advanced and has finally come to a point at which it no longer laughs at the use of color to help heal an individual. Even doctors know that different colors affect their patients in different ways. Blue does indeed make you "blue." Peach or pink encourage people to eat. Do boring work in a red room, wear yellow if you're depressed or black to be less visible.

Color therapy is a useful adjunct to herbal and aroma therapy. Modern mothers will find it very useful when they dress their children or furnish the child's room or paint it. Cooler colors will encourage a very active child to "cool out" while a somber child will be stimulated by more warm and active colors such as tangerine or red. There are many more examples, but try some of the methods that follow and you will be surprised and amazed at the results.

COLOR THERAPY AND AROMATHERAPY THROUGHOUT THE YEAR

JANUARY (CAPRICORN)

Indigo, a dark color, is a combination of very deep blue and violet and of all the colors. Roland Hunt, a pioneer in color therapy, calls indigo unique because it embraces all the colors (the three primaries as well as the three secondaries), and is the "Threshold into the New. It functions as a harmonizer, bringing all together and so in healing it is useful as a purifier, bringing into harmony all the parts of the body." Indigo has power over the Sixth Chakra, considered to be the pineal gland or the third eye. This color and its matching essences (that is, the Balsams, such as Tolu or Peru, and the herb oils, such as Lavender, and the root scents, such as Ginseng) are used for treating the sense organs. This may sound extremely esoteric and to some even ridiculous but color therapy and aromatherapy have been in use for thousands of years as a healing force for the body. In any treatment it is well to use whatever is at hand as well as a combination of treatments rather than just one. So, after your overindulgence during the Christmas holidays, use the simple methods of drinking herb teas, absorbing aromatic oils inhaled through a vaporizer, and thinking and wearing certain colors to purify and heal your body.

Take a piece of indigo-colored silk and spray on Lavender oil. Drape this over your body, especially over the eyes, ears, nose, and throat area. Then lie on a slant board and *think* indigo and *inhale* indigo. Relax, for this meditation will have a soothing, relaxing effect on the body. As you breathe, draw the color thought and scent down into your body into whatever organ is out of whack. Concentrate on the color, wrapping it around the troublesome organ and drawing out impurities and bringing balance to your body. This is called color breathing and if done every day reinforces your powers of positive thinking and can indeed create a healing climate within the body.

Burn the heavy resinous oils such as Tolu, Peru, and even the herby Lavender oil in a container or drop the oils on a lit light bulb. The oil will vaporize and scent the room, purifying the air. You can also put a few drops of the oil into the well of a vaporizer and let the hot, moist steam carry the scent throughout your home or office. These oils are useful as antiseptics and when you breathe them they have a soothing, healing effect on the respiratory system.

Soothing and rather sedative, like their relationship to the color indigo, the oils can be very relaxing and aid in bringing on sleep. So throw away your sleeping pills, drink a cup of Lavender tea, burn the essential oils in a vaporizer, and make your bed up with indigo-colored sheets; these will certainly be a more effective and tranquil means of getting a satisfying night's sleep than any pill. They also create a pleasant and purifying climate in which to rest.

FEBRUARY (AQUARIUS)

Blue is our color. It is cooling and calming. It reduces hot inflammation. Sensitive, high-strung, nervous people should always use blue cotton or flannel sheets to sleep between. Blue, blue, the color of Borage blossom, the color of a bright blue sky on a spring morning or the color of the blue tooth in Jeanne Rose's mouth.

In a passion of hippy madness one spring day in 1969, I forced my conservative dentist to make a blue porcelain tooth to be inserted into a hole left by a previous dentist who cared only for gassing me for giggles rather than repairing holey teeth. I chose the blue color to represent the blue of the sky, to keep me calm (I am normally very much the opposite, being of Latin temperament), so that I could see the color whenever I brushed my teeth, and to keep my spirits light and airy (I am prone to rootedness, being of sanguine temperament).

Blue is the color of the Fifth Chakra (the energy center located in the region of the throat). Blue is astringent and reduces agitation and even bleeding. It has action on the thyroid and the thymus. You can eat blue by eating blueberries; think blue; drink blue, such as the tea that is made from Blue Malva flowers; feel "blue," that is, sad; breathe blue-scented air, that is, blue silk cloths draped over the body that have been scented with flower oils, such as Violet flowers, or resins like Myrrh, Frankincense, or Spikenard. These aromas are quieting, astringent, and antiseptic. They can be used for wounds, coughs, or flatulence.

MARCH (PISCES)

Our color is *purple* and our scent is that of the Violet and the white Narcissus. There is a mystery and wisdom in color-healing and color-breathing not readily apparent. The first step in healing is the effort of the inner self, the ego, to hold itself "erect" in the environment. By awakening yourself to colors and to scents, you will begin to awaken to the world in a new and helpful way. Rudolf Steiner says that the soul lives and rejoices in color and exalts in scent. It is said that flowers emit their fragrance in music or as music while manifesting their selves as color.

These are delightful concepts that should be pursued individually. A "down-to-earth" way to get involved with the concepts of color therapy and aromatherapy is to go outside at any time of the year and sit before a plant. *Look* at it and observe its color; then *smell* it carefully and slowly. The first scent of the volatile oils as they drift off into the atmosphere and into the mucous membranes of your nose is its perfume or fragrance. As you smell more deeply you will "get" the scent of the leaves, the stem, the deeper, more resonating qualities of the "perfume." Now *listen* to the plant and you may hear its low murmuring hum. This sound is their music.

Purple is a royal shade, signifying majesty and rulers. It is of the highest color vibration, a color of strength and power. The person who develops purple in his or her aura can hold responsibility for the care of large numbers of people. Purple is a vascular stimulant, a Piscean color; it increases the functional activity of the kidneys, is an agent in the healing of malaria, lowers the blood pressure and temperature, seems to decrease sexual desires, builds sexual powers by lowering sensitivity, decreases sensitivity to pain, acts as a nerve soother and sleep inducer, and increases the ability to meditate. Leonardo da Vinci said that one could meditate ten times better under violet light streaming through stained-glass windows of a quiet church. Wagner used purple velvet curtains hanging about the area when he composed his music. Babies sleep more gently when put under Violet-scented purple silk cloths.

Violet scent is used in the same way as the purple color. Use color and scent together to effect greater changes.

APRIL (ARIES)

Our color is *scarlet* and our scents are those of the Red Carnation, the Red Rose *(Rosa gallica),* and the pungent Garlic. Flowers that are small and light red are indicated now. Using scarlet or light red as a garment or covering increases activity of the arteries, kidneys, reproductive organs, and emotions. Remember the phrase "to see red"? Red blankets can be emmenagogic when used for an amenorrheic condition. It can be used as an aphrodisiacal color: the red light used to distinguish a house of prostitution.

In color therapy red is often used to balance the functions of the sex organs and to disperse congestion. Many books suggest that women having menstrual difficulties should use light red cotton flannel or wool blankets to bring on the period and blue ones to stop it; this might also be a good suggestion for the pubescent girl.

Jasmine is a soothing scent used to stimulate the sexual organs and to relax the senses. When rubbed on the temples it relieves headache. Jasmine is one of the oils I always carry in my Scentual First-Aid kit, and I have demonstrated its efficacy in the relief of head pains on many occasions. The Jasmine flower itself is either white or light scarlet and its scent is considered to vibrate in red color. So it fits in well with our color-scent correlations.

Fresh Marjoram herb is delicious on Tomatoes and salads, and as a sleep aid its essential oil can be rubbed on the body or inhaled. The herb Hops can be stuffed into a pillow and slept upon for restful sleep.

MAY (TAURUS)

Now is the time to eat blossoms: eating Carnations helps the muscles and sinews; Borage blossoms contain calcium, as do Comfrey blossoms; Rosemary blossoms both relax and stimulate. The blossom can be added to salads or eaten as is and, of course, the scents are very soothing to the spirit. Rubbing a pure oil of Jasmine blossom on the temples can quickly eliminate a headache, while Sage oil rubbed into the neck is an added benefit along with a neck and shoulder massage. The perfumes of Taurus are all the Rose scents, while the flowers are all the spring flowers.

Surround yourself with the colors of spring—pastels, yellow, and light blue. Frames covered with yellow silk and placed between your body and the sun are considered to be a nerve builder, and I have used this method along with color-solarized-fragrance-fans to remove the pain of sciatica. Blue is very calming and can be used alternately with yellow.

Herbal BodyWorks in San Francisco sells potpourris that combine color and (natural, not synthetic) fragrance therapy. A yellow-solarized-fragrance-fan can be made by sandwiching a yellow vibratory potpourri called Verbena potpourri between layers of yellow silk. An ounce of this mixture will emit a Verbena fragrance that is very refreshing and useful for stress and to help the nerves.

Yellow is the color emphasized this month. Yellow stimulates the Third Chakra, the one located in the region of the solar plexus and considered to be the brain of the nervous system. Yellow purifies the system through its eliminative action on the liver and intestines; it has a cleansing and healing effect on the skin through its action on the pores. Yellow is a muscle stimulant, a nerve builder. It is an optimistic color; it is cheering. It is considered a useful color for mental pursuits. It can also be injurious and overexciting to an active system.

In my life yellow has had a very negative effect. Chrome yellow used to be the color of my kitchen, the lower part of the wall was chrome orange. While these nerve colors stimulated my artist husband (now no longer with me) to great creative endeavors they only made me nervous and fidgety and I never could stay in the kitchen for very long. (Maybe that is why I never cooked much, nor did the dishes—although he was quite adequate at dish-washing and became reasonable at cooking). As soon as I realized the problem, I divorced him (my fourth such) and repainted the kitchen mauve and rose and now it is for me a much more relaxing and comfortable place to be. I even cook and wash dishes on occasion.

Yellow foods are Parsnips, Yellow Peppers, Corn, Yams, Yellow Tomatoes, Pineapples, Bananas, Lemons, and other yellow-skinned fruits and vegetables. Scents that vibrate yellow are the Wallflower, Lemon Verbena, Orris root, Cassia, Calamus, and Acacia.

JUNE (GEMINI)

Magenta and the scent of Lilac and Lavender are the scents and color of the season. It is interesting to note that both Lilac and Lavender are indeed almost magenta in color. Rarely do the name of the color and the name of the scent so closely correspond. Magenta is made by combining red and violet. We can say that it is what connects the beginning and the end of the rainbow. The color is used for ailments in the heart area. Green balances and tonifies while magenta heals. Since at this time of the year we are learning about scents from all the blooming flowers, it follows that we should clear and cleanse the respiratory system, including the bronchii. Magenta has been used for this purpose. Earlier we spoke of color-healing using thought and concentration on the color. Remember the exercise: Draw in the color magenta through the air passages, passing it over the entire breathing system for its healing value. Dinshah, a color expert and author, states that magenta is useful as a general stimulant for the entire body, energizing the heart, and as a stabilizer for the emotions. It is also used to build a healthy aura.

While we use magenta in color therapy we can use Peppermint in Aromatherapy. To combine these 2 esoteric therapies simply scent a piece of magenta silk with oil of Peppermint. Lie down with the silk near the head and concentrate on the color magenta while you breathe in the fumes of the Peppermint. As magenta is used for the respiratory system, so the scent Peppermint, a yang scent, is used for clearing and cleansing. Peppermint is an important oil therapeutically. Its taste and odor are familiar to all of us. It is an analgesic and a sedative, cooling to a hot fever, and has great value in all sorts of respiratory conditions, such as colds, flu, or virus infections. It cools by constricting the capillaries and can be used cosmetically as a skin tonic and in homeopathic remedies for various viral and fungal diseases, such as ringworm, shingles, and scabies.

Lilac and Lavender scent are useful for their action on the head and heart. Robert Tisserand mentions that Lavender "has a sedative and tonic action on the heart (hysteria, nervous tension, palpitations) and lowers high blood pressure. It is a mild local analgesic, and calms cerebro-spinal excitability; it is renowned for its nervine-sedative properties, and has proved valuable in a variety of nervous and psychological disorders."

The essential oils can be used in baths, on properly coordinated color screens, as massage oils, or in acupressure massage.

JULY (CANCER)

Green is the color and Anise, Tuberose, and Orange flower the scent. Green is the color of the heart chakra, the color of Vivaldi's music. Surround yourself with green color, green sounds, green foods, and green scents. This total environment will help to balance your energy and bring you to tranquility. Think of a green meadow, the soft green grass in the morning when the dew is still on the blades, a dark green forest, and the soft sea green of the ocean. Green is sedative, relaxing, softly rhythmic. Green energizes the heart, restores rhythm to the system, and strengthens the nerves. Green brings peace and rest. Green is the color of Nature. Ouseley says it "is a soothing harmonious radiation that is essential for the well-being of our nerves and the proper functioning for the body." Green in any form is a tonic to tired nerves and is used for diseases of the heart and blood and the nerves in the head. It restores balance. It is a good idea to use the color green in conjunction with appropriate music, such as Vivaldi's *Four Seasons,* and to have a diffusor in the room that contains Anise oil or Orange flower oil. These oils when vaporized add to the healthful, tonic effect of the color. My living room is painted a clear, rich green, the trim is off-white, and the furnishings are all wicker and wood. This room provides a peaceful, healthful respite for all who walk into it. It is a wonderful, healing reading room.

Green stimulates the pituitary, releases tension, brings blood pressure up or down to normal; relieves head colds and hay fever and asthma; and is thought by some to be the color of vitamin B_1. Green is called the Master Healer.

Thus the combination of green color with Orange flower scent and Vivaldi music is especially healing and particularly efficacious in restoring balance and harmony to a household.

AUGUST (LEO)

The color now is *orange*. Orange gives energy. It also has a mental quality. The fragrance of orange is the perfume of the Orange blossom, the Vanilla orchid, the Bergamot Orange, and the flowers of this time are all the lovely golden ones and the very deep yellow blossoms.

Orange color stimulates the thyroid and the mammary glands, and increases secretions. It is warming, nonastringent, and cheering. It controls the Second Chakra, located in the sacral region. It is symbolic of courage and is the emotional color of worry. Orange is the color of calcium. It is a body normalizer, used to treat asthma, to balance the function of the thyroid, to normalize calcium absorption, to release nervous tension, and to improve digestion and assimilation. It works directly on the spleen and the intestine.

Orange should be used with discrimination; too much of it inclines one to overindulging, not only in food but also in concepts and ideas.

Don't use harsh yellow or orange in the kitchen. It can cause nervous indigestion. My kitchen was chrome yellow and pure orange for years until my divorce, when I painted it mauve and rose. I noticed that my temperament changed from the franticness of the yellow to the calm of the blue within the mauves.

Orange foods are Apricots, Carrots, Eggs, all the lovely Melons that are now in season, and Pumpkins. These all contain vitamin A in abundance and are used for the health of mucous membranes, including those within the intestine. Eat the orange foods, such as Carrots and Oranges, and interpose Vanilla- or Bergamot-scented orange-colored silk screens between the sun and your body to revive you when your energy is low. Since arthritis is partly a problem of calcium absorption, soft orange flannel sheets help correct this disorder.

Orange therapy is used as a body normalizer, fosters optimism, helps the digestion and the assimilation of new ideas, and induces enlightenment and a sense of freedom from limitation.

The Orange blossom is used for depression and hysteria. The oil called Neroli is distinctly soothing and anti-inflammatory to the skin. It seems especially useful in cosmetic creams and treatments for dry skin and, Tisserand says, "it is one of the oils which acts on a cellular level, stimulating the elimination of old cells and the growth of new ones."

Orange flower water has a gentle, soothing effect on children. It can be used as a sedative; a few teaspoons of Orange flower water added to Coffee moderates the jangling effect of the caffeine. If you like to drink this herbal brew but you don't want your hands to shake then just add the Orange flower water to every cup of Coffee that you drink.

Orange flower or Neroli oil is used for its antidepressant, antiseptic, cordial, digestive, and sedative properties. Orange flower water added to Coffee will take away the jittery effect that Coffee often brings. Of course, it would be better to stop drinking Coffee, but if you like the stimulation but not the jitters then add a teaspoon of Orange flower water to every cup you drink. Neroli oil, extracted from the flowers of the bitter Orange tree, *Citrus vulgaris,* has been used for centuries as a perfume for the body, the bath, and clothing. It is considered one of the rejuvenative and regenerative oils. Massaged into the temples it calms the mad pace of a busy mind. It is also used in massage as a treatment for all kinds of skin problems, stimulating the elimination of dead cells and the growth of new ones.

SEPTEMBER (VIRGO)

This is the month of the color violet or dark violet. Violet stimulates the spleen and the building of white blood cells, builds resistance, regulates tension of blood vessels, lowers high blood pressure, slightly depresses the heart, and depresses the lymphatic system. Violet depresses and relaxes the nerves and any overactive part of the body. It can depress the appetite and give relief to an overactive digestive system. This is especially important during the holidays and during vacation time when we all have a tendency to overeat. To use violet color therapy for relaxation, make a mixture of powdered Cinnamon bark, Cloves, and Sandalwood. Enclose this mixture in a sack. Place this sack on a violet-colored silken cloth and the cloth on your body and lie in the sun. The color, the sun, and the scent will soothe an irritated digestive system. You could also put the sack of herbs into a shallow bath with the silk cloth (to incorporate the scent into the color). After it is wet, let dry and the cloth will have a lovely scent. As you lie in the sun with the colored, scented herbs on your body, the breeze will lift the delicious, soothing scent to your nostrils.

Herbs and plants that are considered violet in their color nature are Clovers, Carnations, Rosemary, Cinnamon, and Violets. These are generally yang herbs of very stimulating nature. For instance, the Carnation plant is comforting and releases erotic tension. Use Carnation oil as a massage to tone up the uterus and surrounding muscles. (As an aside, note that Carnation and Rosemary, which are both violet in their color nature, are specifics for the muscular system. Carnation can affect the heart directly in a romantic sense as well as through the sex organs. Carnation's fragrance is violet, although its petal color is pink, red, or white.)

Peppermint stimulates. It affects the brain. It is very useful for the digestive system; its properties are antispasmodic, carminative, cordial, and expectorant, and it reduces fever. It also helps the liver, stomach, and gall bladder. The oil is of great use therapeutically and its refreshing, cooling nature is familiar to all of us. It can be used directly on the skin to relieve itching or irritation, or mixed with oils for a scabies and ringworm deterrent. Homeopathically, Peppermint is used to treat shingles.

Spray the oil on violet-colored paper for use as stationery or on cloth or violet sheets to combine the treatments of color therapy and aromatherapy.

OCTOBER (LIBRA)

Lemon yellow is an alterative, that is, it is an agent that produces gradual beneficial change in the body without any marked specific effect. It is a thymus activator, a laxative, and an expectorant. It is also considered to be a bone-builder and can be used in much the same way as orange color. Lemon yellow sheets would be a helpful adjunct to the therapy used for a bad back. Lemon yellow can act as a blood purifier and apparently loosens and eliminates mucus throughout the body, thus effectively relieving colds. A good scent to use with lemon color is Galbanum, as an incense, as well as the essential oil of Bergamot *(Citrus bergamia)*. When mixed with carrier oils the scent is soothing and the oil healing. This mixture can be used as a massage oil over the lower back and abdominal area to soothe the excretory system. Rosemary, Lavender, and Basil are useful for the bones, joints, and muscles, and be used directly with acupressure to stimulate deeply irritated or sensitive muscles.

NOVEMBER (SCORPIO)

Red is the first color of the spectrum, the color of Scorpio, of blood, of activity and adventure. Corinne Helene says that red is the dominant decorative motif of most primitive people. It is the antidote to fear, to timidity; it is the dominant color of sex or of the bordello—that is, of sexual excitement. In excess it is a sign of danger, as in the red stop sign. It is a physically stimulating color. It energizes the bloodstream and the liver. It is a sensory stimulant and blood builder. Red is an elementary color. Red light builds up plants, then turns them back into the soil, red-solarized water or food controls the First Chakra, which is at the base of the spine. This chakra controls the generative organs as well as the ductless glands to release adrenaline. Red color treatments release, expand, and provide warmth. Red sheets can be used as a menstrual aid by young girls who are having their menstrual cycle and need to allow their bodies to release the menstrual fluids. Red treatments are used for skin disease. Red brings boils and pustules to a head. Red is the color of life, strength, and vitality, as well as of fear.

Red is the color, Rose is the scent. Real red, deep, rich red and lovely Rose scent. Rose-scented red color helps ruptures, uterine problems, and depression.

The scent of red is the scent that is released from the Rose, Geranium, and Jasmine. If possible, keep these perfumes and essential oils in red containers to fix and hold their scent. Roses as well as their essential oils are used as antidepressants and tonics for the entire system. Rose and Jasmine are useful to relieve headaches, whether you take the Rose as tea or use the Jasmine oil to massage on the temples. Red and Rose-scented fans increase the blood pressure and improve circulation. Rose oil mixed with Sandalwood oil and released through the air by placing the oil on the blades of an electric fan is mildly aphrodisiacal. Dim red lights will heighten the mood even further. Roses have been used to treat venereal disease, although this is no longer considered an effective remedy. Rose oil in cosmetics works especially well on dry or mature skin.

Use the oil from the red Rose in massage oils and medicinal oils (commercially, Rose oil comes from the white Rose rather than the Red). Scent a piece of red silk with a red Rose potpourri or Rose oil, lay the silk on your generative organs, lie down in the cool autumn sun, and feel how your reproductive center is charged with energy. Burn incense such as Opopanax at the same time for a complete aromatherapy treatment.

When shopping for aromas always go in the late afternoon, as your sense of smell is sharpest later in the day. Women should not buy scented items during their menstrual period because their sense of smell is somewhat distorted at this time. If you are planning to have an aroma/memory event do it late in the evening when the light is dim and your sense of smell is most perceptive. Scent is very individualistic and mixes with your own body oils to produce a very personal fragrance. Your scent is as much your own as your fingerprints.

Aromatherapy, like color therapy, can be totally personalized, taking into account the uses of the color and scent and where you want to make changes in your body.

DECEMBER (SAGITTARIUS)

December's color is *turquoise*. Its flowers are from flowering trees and climbing vines. The aroma vibrating in the turquoise color is violet, and the gemstone is the turquoise so valued by the Navahoes. The color turquoise is a combination of blue and green, having the qualities of both colors. It is considered a cerebral depressant, decreasing the functional activity of the brain. A powerful alterative, it produces a favorable change in the body through the nutritional processes. It is a skin-builder and superb tonic to the system. The herb Violet, as well as its scent when used aromatherapeutically, also has these qualities. The gemstone turquoise is considered an alterative stone, especially in the nutrition of the body. It strengthens the eyes and protects against accidental falls or violent death. I suppose that if one had a statue of Saint Barbara (the patron saint and protectress of those in danger of dying suddenly, without the sacraments) that was carved in turquoise, resting on a piece of Violet-scented turquoise-colored cloth, one would have a very powerful talisman against sudden or violent death.

The three therapies should be brought together—aromatherapy using Violent scent, gem therapy using the turquoise, and color therapy using turquoise color—to form a powerful force in keeping healthy and well.

Use color and scent to treat all sorts of objects around the home from stationery paper and bookmarks to gems and shells and even lingerie. I like to put small seashells scented with appropriate scents in drawers and jewelry boxes to scent the clothes and the various necklaces and earrings. You can mix any combination of oils, depending on what effect you want. A mixture that seems particularly efficacious is one of Bergamot, Sandalwood, Lavender, and Rose, plus a dab of civet if available. These oils or pomades can be mixed in various quantities. Dip cotton balls in this mixture and stuff the balls into small shells. Store the shells in a tightly closed container. When dry, use the shells in any container to perfume its contents.

Glossary of Words Used in Herbal Health

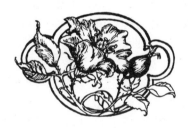

Alterative: An agent that produces gradual beneficial change in the body, usually by improving nutrition, without having any marked specific effect and without causing sensible evacuation.

Analgesic: A drug that relieves or diminishes pain; anodyne.

Anaphrodisiac: An agent that reduces sexual desire or potency.

Anesthetic: An agent that deadens sensation.

Anodyne: An agent that soothes or relieves pain.

Anthelmintic: An agent that destroys or expels intestinal worms; vermicide; vermifuge.

Antibiotic: An agent that destroys or arrests the growth of micro-organisms.

Anticoagulant: An agent that prevents clotting in a liquid, as in blood.

Antiemetic: An agent that counteracts nausea and relieves vomiting.

Antihydrotic: An agent that reduces or suppresses perspiration.

Antiperiodic: An agent that counteracts periodic or intermittent diseases (such as malaria).

Antipyretic: An agent that prevents or reduces fever.

Antiseptic: An agent for destroying or inhibiting pathogenic or putrefactive bacteria.

Antispasmodic: An agent that relieves or checks spasms or cramps.

Aperient: A mild stimulant for the bowels; a gentle purgative.

Aphrodisiac: An agent for arousing or increasing sexual desire or potency.

Appetizer: An agent that excites the appetite.

Aromatic: A substance having an agreeable odor and stimulating qualities.

Astringent: An agent that contracts organic tissue, reducing secretions or discharges.

Balsam: 1) A soothing or healing agent. 2) a resinous substance obtained from the exudations of various trees and used in medicinal preparations.

Bitter: Characterized by a bitter principle that acts on the mucous membranes of the mouth and stomach to increase appetite and promote digestion.

Calmative: An agent that has a mild sedative or tranquilizing effect.

Cardiac: An agent that stimulates or otherwise affects the heart.

Carminative: An agent for expelling gas from the intestines.

Cathartic: An agent that acts to empty the bowels; laxative.

Cholagogue: An agent for increasing the flow of bile into the intestines.

Coagulant: An agent that induces clotting in a liquid, as in blood.

Counterirritant: An agent for producing irritation in one part of the body to counteract irritation or inflammation in another part.

Demulcent: A substance that soothes irritated tissue, particularly mucous membrane.

Deodorant: An herb that has the effect of destroying or masking odors.

Depressant: An agent that lessens nervous or functional activity; opposite of stimulant.

Depurative: An agent that purifies the system, particularly the blood.

Detergent: An agent that cleanses wounds and sores of diseased or dead matter.

Diaphoretic: An agent that promotes perspiration; sudorific.

Digestive: An agent that promotes or aids digestion.

Diuretic: An agent that increases the secretion and expulsion of urine.

Emetic: An agent that causes vomiting.

Emmenagogue: An agent that promotes menstrual flow.

Emollient: An agent used externally to soften and soothe.

Expectorant: An agent that promotes the discharge of mucus from the respiratory passages.

Febrifuge: An agent that reduces or eliminates fever.

Fomentation: Cloths soaked in hot herbal decoctions or infusions and wrung out and applied to sore, infected, or aching areas to reduce inflammation or ease pain.

Hemostatic: An agent that stops bleeding.

Hepatic: A drug that acts on the liver.

Hydragogue: A purgative that produces abundant water discharge.

Hypnotic: An agent that promotes or produces sleep.

Infusion: A mixture of herb and water, brought to a boil, removed from the fire, steeped or infused, and used as a drink or an external wash.

Irritant: An agent that causes inflammation or abnormal sensitivity in living tissue.

Laxative: An agent promoting evacuation of the bowels; a mild purgative.

Macerate: To extract and soften by soaking in a fluid.

Mucilaginous: Characterized by a gummy or gelatinous consistency.

Nephritic: A medicine applicable to diseases of the kidney.

Nervine: An agent that has a calming or soothing effect on the nerves; formerly, any agent that acts on the nervous system.

Oxytocic: An agent that stimulates contraction of the uterine muscle and so facilitates or speeds up childbirth.

Pectoral: A remedy for pulmonary or other chest diseases.

Poultice: An application of hot, moist herb or infusion directly to the skin.

Purgative: An agent that produces a vigorous emptying of the bowels.

Restorative: An agent that restores consciousness or normal physiological activity.

Rubefacient: A gentle local irritant that produces reddening of the skin.

Sedative: A soothing agent that reduces nervousness, distress, or irritation.

Sialagogue: An agent that stimulates the secretion of saliva.

Specific: An agent that cures or alleviates a particular condition or disease.

Stimulant: An agent that excites or quickens the activity of physiological processes.

Stomachic: An agent that strengthens, stimulates, or tones the stomach.

Styptic: An agent that contracts tissues; astringent; specifically, a hemostatic agent that stops bleeding by contracting the blood vessels.

Sudorific: An agent that promotes or increases perspiration.

Tincture: A strained solution of herbs and alcohol, to be used internally or externally.

Tonic: An agent that strengthens or invigorates organs or the entire organism.

Vasoconstrictor: An agent that narrows the blood vessels, thus raising blood pressure.

Vasodilator: An agent that widens the blood vessels, thus lowering blood pressure.

Vermicide: An agent that destroys intestinal worms.

Vermifuge: An agent that causes the expulsion of intestinal worms.

Vesicant: An agent that produces blisters.

Vulnerary: A healing application for wounds.

Bibliography

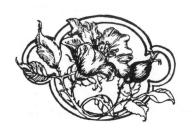

Anderson, Edgar, *Plants, Man and Life*. Berkeley: University of California Press, 1969.

Clarkson, Rosetta E., *Herbs, Their Culture and Uses*. New York: The Macmillan Publishing Co., 1968.

Davis, Adelle, *Let's Have Healthy Children*. New York: Harcourt Brace, Jovanovitch, Inc., 1951.

Gerarde, *The Herbal or General History of Plants*, 2 vol. London: Adan, Islip, Joice Norton and Richard Whitakers, 1636.

Glas, Norbert, M.D., *Conception, Birth and Early Childhood*. Spring Valley, NY: Anthroposophic Press, Inc., 1972.

Grieve, Mrs. M., *A Modern Herbal*. New York: Hafner Publishing Co., 1971.

Hunt, Roland T., *The Seven Keys to Color Healing*. London: The C.W. Daniel Co., 1971.

Koehler, Nan, *Artemis Speaks: VBAC Stories and Natural Childbirth Information*. Occidental, CA: Jerald R. Brown, Inc., 1985.

Lappe, Frances Moore, *Diet for a Small Planet*. New York: Ballantine Books, 1971.

Leyel, Mrs. C. F., *The Magic of Herbs*. London: Jonathon Cape, 1926.

Maury, Marguerite, *The Secret of Life and Youth*. London: Macdonald, 1964.

McNair, James, *The World of Herbs and Spices*. San Francisco, CA: Ortho Books, 1978.

Messegue, Maurice, *Way to Natural Health and Beauty*. New York: The Macmillan Publishing Co., 1974.

Popov, Ivan, M.D., *Stay Young*. New York: Grosset & Dunlap, 1975.

Robertson, Laurel, Carol Flinders, and Bronwen Godfrey, *Laurel's Kitchen: A Handbook for Vegetarian Cookery and Nutrition*. New York: Bantam Books, 1978.

Rose, Jeanne, *Herbs & Things*. New York: Grosset & Dunlap, 1972.

———, *Jeanne Rose's Herbal Body Book*. New York: Grosset & Dunlap, 1976.

———, *Kitchen Cosmetics*. San Francisco, CA: Panjandrum Books, 1978.

———, *Jeanne Rose's Herbal Guide to Inner Health*. New York: Grosset & Dunlap, 1979.

Tisserand, Robert B., *The Art of Aromatherapy*. The C. W. Daniel Co., Ltd., 1977.

Wood, George B., M.D., and Franklin Bache, M.D., *The Dispensatory of the U.S.A.* Philadelphia: J. B. Lippincott & Co., 1873.

zur Linden, Wilhelm, *A Child Is Born*. London; Rudolph Steiner Press, 1973.

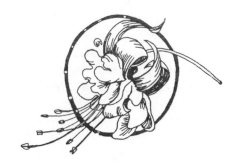

Index

• • •

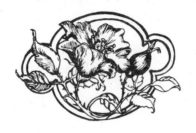

If you enjoyed this book,
you'll also want to order

Jeanne Rose's Herbal Body Book
ISBN 0-399-50790-6
The herbal way to natural beauty and health for
men and women.

Herbs and Things
ISBN 0-399-50944-5
Eating right the herbal way,
with more than 120 recipes.

For your convenience, use the coupon to order.
Attach an additional page if necessary.
These books are also available at your local bookstore
or wherever paperback books are sold.

G. P. Putnam's Sons
390 Murray Hill Parkway, Dept. B
East Rutherford, New Jersey 07073

Please send me _____ copies of *Jeanne Rose's Herbal Body
Book* (SBN 399-50790-6) at $9.95 each.

Please send me _____ copies of *Herbs and Things*
(SBN 399-50944-5) at $8.95 each.

Enclosed is my ☐ check ☐ money order. Please charge my ☐ Visa ☐ MasterCard. Card # _____ Expiration date _____	Subtotal $ _____ Postage & Handling $ _1.50_ Sales Tax $ _____ **Total** $ _____

Name _____

Address_____

City _____ State ____ Zip ____

Signature as on charge card _____

Please allow 4 to 6 weeks for delivery.

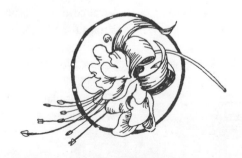